Topics in
Gastroenterology
8

This book is dedicated to

MRS. ZENA JENNINGS

in recognition of her invaluable services in
the organisation of the annual postgraduate courses
on which this series is based

Topics in Gastroenterology
8

EDITED BY
S. C. TRUELOVE
MA, MD, FRCP

AND
H. J. KENNEDY
MB, BS, MRCP

BLACKWELL SCIENTIFIC PUBLICATIONS
OXFORD LONDON EDINBURGH
BOSTON MELBOURNE

© 1980 by
Blackwell Scientific Publications
Editorial offices:
Osney Mead, Oxford, OX2 0EL
8 John Street, London, WC1N 2ES
9 Forrest Road, Edinburgh, EH1 2QH
52 Beacon Street, Boston
    Massachusetts 02108, USA
214 Berkeley Street, Carlton
    Victoria 3053, Australia

First published 1980

Set by Express Litho Service (Oxford)
Printed and bound in Great Britain
by the Alden Press Ltd
Oxford

DISTRIBUTORS
USA
    Blackwell Mosby Book Distributors
    11830 Westline Industrial Drive
    St Louis, Missouri 63141

Canada
    Blackwell Mosby Book Distributors
    120 Melford Drive, Scarborough
    Ontario, M1B 2X4

Australia
    Blackwell Scientific Book Distributors
    214 Berkeley Street, Carlton
    Victoria 3053

British Library
Cataloguing in Publication Data

Topics in Gastroenterology
    8.
    1. Gastroenterology — Periodicals
    I. Truelove, S.C.
    II. Kennedy, H.J.
    616.3   RC816

ISBN 0-632-00725-7

Contents

Treatment of Crohn's Disease

Some Aspects of Ulcerative Colitis

Miscellaneous Topics

Preface

As with previous volumes in this series, this book is a written version of the annual course in gastroenterology held in January of the current year. It is a great pleasure to thank our contributors whose chapters are based on the lectures they gave in the course.

We are grateful to our publishers, Blackwell Scientific Publications, and in particular to Mr Per Saugman, their Chairman and Managing Director, and to Mr John Robson, their Production Director, with whom it is a pleasure to co-operate.

Nuffield Department of Clinical Medicine   S. C. Truelove
University of Oxford   H. J. Kennedy

Contributors

Mr. R. M. Baddeley, *General Hospital, Steelhouse Lane, Birmingham.*

Professor J. C. Goligher, *Glebe House, 5 Shaw Lane, Leeds.*

Dr. M. J. Goodman, *Bury General Hospital, Bury, Lancs.*

Mr. Graham L. Hill, *University Department of Surgery, General Infirmary, Leeds.*

Dr. D. P. Jewell, *John Radcliffe Hospital, Oxford.*

Mr. Peter F. Jones, *Woodend General Hospital, Aberdeen.*

Dr. H. Joyeux, *Centre Anticancereux, Cliniques Saint-Eloi, 34059 Montpellier Cedex, France.*

Miss Penny Kane, *John Radcliffe Hospital, Oxford.*

Mr. M. R. B. Keighley, *General Hospital, Steelhouse Lane, Birmingham.*

Dr. H. J. Kennedy, *John Radcliffe Hospital, Oxford.*

Mr. M. G. W. Kettlewell, *John Radcliffe Hospital, Oxford.*

Professor Nils G. Kock, *University of Göteborg, Sahlgrenska Sjukhuset, S-143 45 Göteborg, Sweden.*

Mr. Emanoel C. G. Lee, *John Radcliffe Hospital, Oxford.*

Professor H. A. Lee, *St. Mary's Hospital, Portsmouth, Hants.*

Professor J. E. Lennard-Jones, *Academic Unit of Gastroenterology, The London Hospital, Whitechapel, London.*

Dr. J. I. Mann, *John Radcliffe Hospital, Oxford.*

Mr. Adrian Marston, *82 Harley Street, London.*

Dr. Jeremy Powell-Tuck, *Clinical Nutrition and Metabolism Unit, Hospital for Tropical Diseases, 4 St. Pancras Way, London.*

Dr. B. D. Ross, *Department of Biochemistry, Radcliffe Infirmary, Oxford.*

Mr. Gavin Royle, *John Radcliffe Hospital, Oxford.*

Professor Cl. Solassol, *Centre Anticancereux, Cliniques Saint-Eloi, 34059 Montpellier Cedex, France.*

Dr. S. C. Truelove, *Radcliffe Infirmary, Oxford.*

Dr. C. P. Willoughby, *John Radcliffe Hospital, Oxford.*

Professor H. F. Woods, *Section of Pharmacology, Hallamshire Hospital, Sheffield.*

Parenteral Feeding

Chapter 1

The development of parenteral nutrition

H. A. LEE

The historical background to parenteral nutrition can be found in reviews by Wilkinson (1963) and Lee (1974). Probably the first attempt at injecting a liquid into the blood stream was made by Dr Robert Boyle in 1659 following a suggestion by Sir Christopher Wren in 1658 that any liquid could be injected into the circulation. Clearly, these ideas arose from the discovery of the circulation by Sir William Harvey in 1625. In 1664 Caspar Scotus injected wine intravenously and then a year later Sir Christopher Wren gave alcohol intravenously. One of the earliest attempts at giving oil intravenously was by Courten in 1679. It is interesting to note that in 1818 James Blundell gave the first successful blood transfusion from one human subject to another.

Probably the first major development in intravenous therapy followed the cholera epidemics of the 1820s and 1830s during which abnormalities in blood chemistry were reported by O'Shaughnessy (1839). As a result of these observations, Dr Latta, a general practitioner working near Leith in Scotland, made up appropriate salt solutions and injected these into stricken cholera patients with considerable success. Then, interestingly, one of the father figures of modern medicine, Claude Bernard, in 1858 recorded his observations on the results of intravenous injection of egg-white into animals. Then, as a result of cholera epidemics, this time in Canada, Hodder (1873) reported his observations following the intravenous injection of milk, the results of which, not too surprisingly, were not very successful. About the same time, Menzel and Perco (1869) carried out comprehensive experiments on animals to which they gave subcutaneous injections of mixtures of oil, beaten eggs, sugar solutions and milk, culminating with the injection of such a mixture into an emaciated patient suffering from Pott's disease. The first report in which glucose was used as a source of calories was published in 1899 by Lillienfeld who found that glucose injected intravenously was safe. It fell to Frederich of Leipzig in 1905 to record for the first time the successful maintenance of nutrition by subcutaneous injections of mixtures of water, salts, carbohydrates, fat and peptones for periods varying between 10 and 14 days.

In the early mid-19th century it had been shown that either the administration, or the withholding, of protein could influence nitrogen balance (Bidder and Schmidt, 1852; Voit, 1866). Abderhalden and Rona (1904) were probably the first to show that enzymatically digested protein yielded a solution of peptides and amino acids that could be given intravenously. Some years later, Henriques and Anderson (1913) succeeded in maintaining normal weight in a goat by infusion of such dialysates.

Since then there has been much experimentation with a variety of hydrolysates derived from lactalbumin, bovine serum protein, human serum albumin and horse fibrin. Latterly, casein hydrolysates have been the most commonly used source of protein for intravenous nitrogen administration. However, the early use of protein hydrolysate solutions intravenously was not without setbacks, particularly from toxic reactions. Also, manufacturing difficulties were experienced initially and it was not until the advent of partial enzymatic hydrolysis of protein that preparations containing amino acids and polypeptides were developed without loss of nutritional value or of any of the so-called essential amino acids. This was followed by the development of partial enzymatic hydrolysis coupled with dialysis to remove the larger polypeptides which cause toxic reactions. As a result, Woodyatt *et al.* (1915) and later Rose (1934) suggested the use of parenteral amino acids as a component part of total parenteral nutrition. It was Elman (1937) in St. Louis, U.S.A., who initiated the modern use of protein preparations for intravenous feeding. Shohl and Blackfan (1940) were the first to use a complete mixture of amino acids. Their solution contained 12 dextro and 13 laevo forms of essential and non-essential amino acids and was a modification of a formula proposed by McCoy *et al.* (1935).

The last twenty-five years have seen the development of the pure L form amino acid solutions. These have the advantage of specificity whereas protein hydrolysates contain a fair amount of peptide nitrogen, amonia and other contaminants. Furthermore, there has been an increasing awareness that synthetic crystalline L amino acid solutions need to be balanced, not only with respect to essential amino acids but also in terms of non-essential nitrogen components.

Likewise, in the last two decades there has been a rationalization of the types of substrate used intravenously as a source of energy. Although many different substrates have been investigated, only two need to be considered in modern total parenteral nutrition, namely, glucose and a fat emulsion, such as soybean oil emulsion. Kerr and Pauly (1942) showed that invert sugar could be used intravenously and Wennig (1955) described the use of intravenous honey. Subsequently, sorbitol, xylitol and fructose have all gone through vogues of fashion in intravenous nutrition regimens (Lee, 1974), but really offer no advantages over the other two substrates. Although glycerol has an equal caloric value to glucose and can be given in dilute solution to man (Bowesman, 1938; Sloviter, 1958), it is a dangerous caloric source with serious side-effects.

Alcohol has had its advocates because of its high caloric value of 7 kcal per gram (Rydberg, 1975) but difficulties have occurred because of its known pharmacological effects. Atwater and Benedict (1896) showed that ethyl alcohol could positively affect nitrogen balance and Rice and Strickler (1952) extensively investigated its clinical use. These observations were further extended by Coates (1972), but in current day intravenous feeding alcohol has little, if any, role to play.

Thus, the past twenty years have seen a prodigious amount of experimental work carried out to make comprehensive intravenous feeding a safe and attainable goal, in both the short-term and long-term management of patients who otherwise could not be maintained in nutritional equilibrium. Estimates of patients requiring nutritional support in hospitals vary from 40–50% (Bistrian *et al.*, 1974, 1976; Hill *et al.*, 1977). However, it is likely that only 5–15% of all such patients actually require aggressive nutritional support and of these only 2–4% will need intravenous feeding. Nevertheless, in this nucleus of patients, intravenous feeding may represent the difference between life and death. Many of the technical problems associated with intravenous feeding have been overcome with such modern developments as better silicone catheters, better understanding of catheter maintenance, and the development of safe constant-volumetric intravenous pumps that can be used both in the hospital and in the home.

Probably the most important aspect of intravenous feeding is to be able to recognize the patient who actually requires this type of nutritional support. Having decided that the need exists, it is then important to ascertain the degree of malnutrition that has occurred. This is necessary, not only for defining the problem, but also to confirm that the treatment given is in fact effective. Table 1.1 shows some of

Table 1.1. *Tests for evidence of malnutrition. A profile based on items 1–6 will give a useful guide to nutritional status*

Factor assessed	Method	Evidence of malnutrition
1. General appearance of patient	Visual assessment	Wasting, Emaciation
2. Body weight in kg and recent loss	Various scales	$> 10\%$
3. Triceps skin fold thickness (TST) (fat energy reserves)	Holtain skin fold calipers	< 10 mm in males < 13 mm in females
4. Mid-arm circumference muscle (MAMC) Muscle protein reserves (MAMC = arm circumf. $- \pi$ TST)	Tape measure in cm	< 23 cm in males < 22 cm in females
5. Serum albumin (visceral protein)	Routine lab. test	< 35 g/l
6. Serum transferrin Complement C_3 } short half life proteins	Routine lab. test	< 2 g/l
7. Retinol binding protein Thyroxine binding pre-albumin } ultra short half life proteins	Special lab. tests	< 40 mg/l < 200 mg/l
8. Urinary hydroxyproline	Special lab. test	↑ Collagen turnover
9. Urinary zinc excretion	Special lab. test	↑ due to muscle and collagen breakdown
10. Lymphopaenia	Routine lab. test	$< 1{\cdot}2 \times 10^9/1$
11. Plasma amino acid profile	Specialized tests	Changing valine/glycine ratio
12. Urine 3-methylhistidine	Specialized tests	Increased muscle breakdown
13. Hair root morphology	Tweezers and microscope	More telogens and dysplastic hairs

the measurements used and how they are interpreted. Furthermore, it is important to appreciate that such measurements can easily be undertaken by junior medical and nursing staff, are reproducible, and do not require expensive or complicated equipment.

Having ascertained that a patient is in need of this form of treatment, then the question of angioaccess is the next important step. Much has been written about the techniques available for gaining angioaccess (Dudrick and Long, 1977; Parsa *et al.*, 1972). Basically, there are two main methods, both of which require meticulous aseptic technique. One can either choose a peripheral site and use a long catheter (Abbott flexible drum catheter) or go centrally, using a percutaneous venous route to gain access to the subclavian vein, either supraclavicularly or infraclavicularly. When this latter technique is combined with subcutaneous tunnelling, the catheter can be left in place for weeks on end. Angioaccess in such patients must be regarded as their lifeline and be cared for appropriately (Phillips, 1976). Each individual will perfect his own technique and it is presumptuous to say that one method is better than another in experienced hands. Furthermore, the development of silicone catheters, which are non-irritant, means that the catheter can be left in place for a long time (Broviac and Scribner, 1974). There is no real justification for using shunts or fistulae.

With the better development of administration lines the need for 'piggy-backing' is avoided and the risk of infection considerably decreased. Initially, half-litre bottles were used but nowadays there is a choice between one litre bottles or using the 'big bag' (2—3 1) system (Cosh *et al.*, 1977). This latter method has been developed principally as a result of the studies of Solassol and Joyeux (1976), working in Montpellier in France. They have shown that all nutritional requirements can be mixed in a single bag, even including a fat emulsion. For those who are sceptical of such an approach, the use of one-litre bottles and special W giving sets (welded units) enables all ingredients to be given through a single catheter. There is general agreement that intravenous feeding lines should be used solely for feeding purposes and not for giving blood or plasma, or for measuring central venous pressure. The care of catheter lines, in particular of the skin around the entry point, has been described in detail by Colley (1977). A comprehensive review of the technical aspects can be found in Parsa *et al.* (1972).

Having recognized the patient who requires intravenous feeding and having gained angioaccess, the problem then is what to give, how much to give, and over what time. Fortunately, there is now some agreement about the nutritional requirements of various categories of patient, as shown in Table 1.2. For energy requirements, many would advocate a 50—50 ratio of glucose and fat for energy provision. However, if a patient is known to be septicaemic, or has a known fat intolerance, then more reliance can be made upon concentrated glucose solutions (40—50%), with or without insulin. If insulin has to be given, it can be added to the bottle, even though some will be lost by adhering to the glass surface. Since the aim is to keep the blood sugar below 10 mmol per litre, more soluble insulin can be added if necessary as boluses. The advantages of using a combined fat and glucose regimen are (a) the provision of each substrate is kept well within an individual's tolerance; for example, for a 70 kg man requiring 3,000 kcal per day, this would mean glucose 0·233 g/kg per hour and fat 0·089 g/kg per hour, (b) the volume is kept small, (c) the osmolar load is minimized, being 129 mOsmol/hr, (d) the percentage of energy provided that is lost in the urine is minimal, being less than 5% and (e) minimal monitoring is required and possibly less soluble insulin required.

As for nitrogen sources, it is now generally agreed that there is no single ideal amino acid solution, but there is a range of solutions all of which are adequate. Indeed, Tweedle *et al.* (1973) showed that some of the more modern synthetic crystalline L amino acid solutions, although better defined and with fewer contaminants, were not more effective in maintaining nitrogen balance than the earlier casein/fibrin hydrolysates. Over the past ten years there has been a proliferation of different amino acid solutions said to be necessary for specific situations, but no great variety is required. Indeed, all that is needed is a high nitrogen source solution providing 16—18 g/l, a maintenance solution providing approximately 10 g/l, possibly a specific solution for liver failure (Aguirre *et al.*, 1976) and a further specific one for paediatric use (Lee, 1979 a and b).

Clearly, total intravenous nutrition must take into account not only energy and nitrogen, but also water, electrolytes, fat-soluble and water-soluble vitamins, trace elements, folic acid and phosphate. Each year more is being learned about the so called micronutrients, so that, although we still do not know the precise requirements, such elements as selenium, zinc, chrome, nickel and others may need to be included (Kay *et al.*, 1976; Shenkin and Wretlind, 1978; Aggett, 1979; Van Rij *et al.*, 1979).

The various ingredients need to be combined in optimum ratios, as suggested in Table 1.3. Just as formerly it was inappropriate to talk about 'a drop of water with a pinch of salt' as intravenous solution,

Table 1.2. *Catabolic rates and estimated requirements*

	Protein g(N.g)/day‡	Energy kcal/day	gN/kg body wt	kcal/kg body wt	kcal/gN*
Apyrexial medical patient	45– 75 (7·2–12)	1500–2000	0·16–0·20	30–37	= 170
Post-operative (uncomplicated)	75–100 (12–16)	2000–3500	0·20–0·22	37–45	= 190
Hypercatabolic e.g. burns	> 100 (> 16)	> 3500	0·22–0·30	46–52	= 210

Notes
1. Wide ranges of requirements for each group accentuating risk of underestimating requirements.
2. 1 g nitrogen $\equiv$ 6·25 g protein $\simeq$ 30 g muscle.
3. Many patients breaking down 20 g nitrogen per day $\simeq$ 0·6 kg muscle – hence potential for rapid wasting.

* Recent evidence suggests that in hypercatabolic and normocatabolic patients that the ratio is lower and higher respectively. (Woolfson, 1979). However, the generally accepted 200:1 ratio meets most requirements.
‡ Best estimated by measuring urinary urea nitrogen (Lee and Hartley, 1975).

Table 1.3. *Basic recommendations for designing a daily intravenous nutritional support regimen*

1. Nitrogen: 0·20–0·24 g/kg body weight.
2. Energy: 40–45 kcal/kg body weight.
3. Nitrogen: energy ratio 1:200 (variable according to catabolic status).
4. Energy derived on 50% basis from glucose and fat emulsion or from glucose/insulin/potassium regimen.
5. Optimal potassium: nitrogen ratio = 5 mmol: 1 g.
6. Optimal magnesium: nitrogen ratio = 0·5 mmol: 1 g.
7. Phosphorus intake: 0·5–0·75 mmol/kg body weight.
8. Water soluble vitamins e.g. thiamin 3–5 mg, riboflavin 4–6 mg, pyridoxine 4–6 mg, ascorbic acid 100 mg, folic acid 5 mg.
9. Vitamin K: 3–5 mg.
10. Adequate electrolyte provision.
11. Essential biological elements, e.g. zinc (50 μmol), copper (5 μmol), manganese (6 μmol).
12. Energy and nitrogen given simultaneously.
13. Essential fatty acids, e.g. linoleic acid 100 mg/kg body weight.
14. Blood or plasma (or HPPF) for immediate restoration of haemoglobin or serum oncotic pressure.
15. Even distribution of infusion over 24 hour periods.
16. Mobilize as soon as possible.

so now one must not fall into the trap of simply talking about 'nitrogen with a little sweetener'.

The list of complications associated with intravenous nutrition is quite formidable (Table 1.4). None the less, with the modern approach, which involves adequate monitoring and the use of a limited number of substrates, all these complications are totally avoidable and the amount of monitoring required not excessive. This is why it is important that this form of treatment should be seen, not as the sole preserve of the specialist, but one to be used by all those who deal with critically ill patients, many of whom may require intravenous feeding. Recent reviews on comprehensive regimens can be found in Lee (1974), Fischer (1976), Dickerson and Lee (1978), Shenkin and Wretlind (1978) and Lee (1979b).

With the critically ill patient, it is important to realize that the

Table 1.4. *Complications of intravenous nutrition*

Disturbance	Potential causal substrate or explanation
Metabolic acidosis: lactic acidosis	Fructose; sorbitol; ethanol-carbohydrate combinations
Hyperosmolar dehydration syndrome	Hypertonic glucose, sorbitol, xylitol
Hyperuricaemia	Fructose; sorbitol; xylitol
Oxalaemia and Oxaluria	? xylitol
Triglyceridaemia	Fructose, sorbitol, xylitol, fat emulsion
Hyperlipidaemia	Fat emulsion, particularly in septicaemia
Essential fatty acid deficiency	Fat-free intravenous regimen
Hypophosphataemia	Phosphorus-free, glucose-only regimens
Folate metabolism disturbances	Ethanol
Hyperammonaemia	Protein hydrolysate solution
Hypoglycaemia	Rebound post-infusion phenomenon
Hypo- and hyper-magnesaemia	Inadequate provision, particularly in gastro-intestinal disease. Excessive administration, particularly if renal function compromised
Anaemia	May be due to deficiencies of iron, folic acid, vitamin B_{12}, copper
Bleeding diathesis	Vitamin K deficiency
Cholestatic hepatitis	Amino acid solution
Altered cerebration	Poorly designed amino acid solutions

Angioaccess complications:
  (i) thrombosis
  (ii) sepsis
  (iii) damage to structures during central venous catheterization (e.g. haematoma, haemorrhage, pneumothorax)
	Hypertonic solutions given peripherally

Fatty liver	Glucose solutions

12 *H. A. Lee*

feeding regime required initially is not necessarily appropriate later and so adjustments may have to be made. The need for such adjustments can be deduced by monitoring the patient. Sometimes a patient may benefit from a combination of intravenous and enteral nutrition and these two nutritional methods should never be regarded as mutually exclusive.

Perhaps the ultimate in parenteral nutrition has been realised with the so-called artificial gut system (Shils, 1975). Patients with massive gastro-intestinal resections as a result of infarction, injury or extensive Crohn's disease can now be maintained for years at a time by total parenteral nutrition. Indeed, much about man's requirements of micro-nutrients has been learned from the study of such patients (Leading Article, Brit. med. J. 1978).

Thus, in 1980, there really cannot be any excuse for a critically ill patient dying of malnutrition, though regrettably this still often occurs. First of all, there must be an awareness of a patient's nutritional needs and the clinician must not feel afraid of resorting to intravenous nutrition. Intravenous nutrition is one of the most promising therapeutic developments of the last two decades and needs to be considered in the treatment of any critically ill patient. Although it is an expensive form of treatment, it reduces morbidity and the length of hospital stay and therefore more than justifies the expense (Leading Article, Brit. med. J. 1979).

References

Abderhalden E. and Rona P. (1904) *Hoppe-Seyler's Z. physiol. Chem.* **42**, 528.

Aggett P.J. (1979) Hospital Update, **98**.

Aguirre A., Funovics J., Wesdorp R.I.C. and Fischer J.E. (1976). In *Total Parenteral Nutrition,* ed. Fischer J.E., Little, Brown and Company, Boston.

Atwater W.O. and Benedict F.G. (1896) *Mem. Natn. Acad. Sci.* **8**, 235.

Bistrian B.R., Blackburn G.L., Hallowell E. and Heddle R. (1974) *J. Amer. med. Ass.* **230**, 858.

Bistrian B.R., Blackburn G.L., Vitale J., Cochran D. and Naylor J. (1976) *J. Amer. med. Ass.* **253**, 1567.

Bowesman C. (1938) *Brit. J. Surg.* **26**, 86.

Broviac J.W. and Scribner B.H. (1974) *Surg. Gynec. Obstet.* **139**, 24.

Coats D.A. (1972). In *Parenteral Nutrition,* ed. Wilkinson A.W. Churchill Livingstone, Edinburgh.

Colley R. (1977). In *Current Concepts in Parenteral Nutrition,* eds. Greep J.M., Soetors P.B., Wesdorp R.I.C., Phaf C.W.R. and Fischer J.E. Martinus Nijhoff, The Hague.

Cosh D.G., West K.R., Thomas M.P. and Sansom L.N. (1977) *Aust. J. Pharm. Sci.* **6**, 97.

Dickerson J.W.T. and Lee H.A. eds. (1978) *Nutrition in the Clinical Management of Disease*. Arnold, London.

Dudrick S.J. and Long J.M. (1977). In *Current Concepts in Parenteral Nutrition*, eds. Greep J.M., Soetors P.B., Wesdorp R.I.C., Phaf C.W.R. and Fischer J.E. Martinus Nijhoff, The Hague.

Elman R. (1937) *Proc. Soc. exp. Biol.* **37**, 437.

Fischer J.E. (1976) *Total Parenteral Nutrition*. Little, Brown and Company, Boston.

Henriques V. and Anderson A.C. (1913) *Hoppe-Seyler's Z. Physiol. Chem.* **42**, 357.

Hill G.L., Blackwell R.L., Pickerford I., Birkinshaw L., Young G.A., Warren J.V., Schorah C.J. and Morgan D.B. (1977) *Lancet*, i, 689.

Kay R.G., Tasman-Jones C., Pybus J., Whiting R. and Black H. (1976) *Ann. Surg.* **183**, 331.

Kerr S.E. and Pauly R.J. (1942) *Surg. Gynec. Obstet.* **74**, 925.

Leading article (1978) *Brit. med. J.* ii, 913.

Leading article (1979) *Brit. med. J.* ii, 1529.

Lee H.A. (1974). In *Parenteral Nutrition in Acute Metabolic Illness*, ed. Lee H.A. Academic Press, London.

Lee H.A. (1979a) *Int. J. Vit. Nutr. Res.* **18**, 45.

Lee H.A. (1979b). In *General Anaesthesia 4e*, eds. Gray T.C., Nunn, J.F. and Utting J.E. Butterworths, London.

Lee H.A. and Hartley T.F. (1975) *Postgrad. med. J.* **51**, 441.

McCoy R.H., Meyer C.E. and Rose W.C. (1935) *J. biol. Chem.* **112**, 283.

Parsa M.H., Ferrer J.M. and Habif D.V. (1972) *Safe Central venous nutrition. Guidelines for prevention and management of complications*. Charles C. Thomas, Springfield, Illinois.

Philips K.J. (1976). In *Total Parenteral Nutrition*, ed. Fischer J.E. Little, Brown and Company, Boston.

Rice C.O. and Strickler J.H. (1952) *Geriatrics*, 7, 232.

Rose W.C. (1934) *Harvey Lect.* **30**, 49.

Rydberg U. (1975). In *Total Parenteral Nutrition. Premises and Promises*, ed. Ghadimi H. Wiley, New York.

Shenkin A. and Wretlind A. (1978) *World Rev. Nutr. Diet.* **28**, 1.

Shils M.E. (1975) *Amer. J. clin. Nutr.* **28**, 1429.

Shohl A.T. and Blackfan K.D. (1940) *J. Nutr.* **20**, 305.

Sloviter H.A. (1958) *J. clin. Invest.* **37**, 619.

Solassol C. and Joyeux H. (1976). In *Total Parenteral Nutrition*, ed. Fischer J.E. Little, Brown and Company, Boston.

Tweedle D.E.F., Spivey J. and Johnston I.D.A. (1973) *Metabolism*, **22**, 173.

Van Rij A.M., Thomson C.D., McKenzie J.M. and Robinson M.F. (1979) *Amer. J. clin Nutr.* **32**, 2076.

Wennig E. (1955) *Klin Wschr.* **67**, 110.

Wilkinson A.W. (1963) *Nutr. et Dieta*, **5**, 295.

Woodyatt R.T., Sansum W.D. and Wilder R.N. (1915) *J. Amer. med. Ass.* **65**, 2067.

Woolfson A.M.J. (1979). In *Developments in Clinical Nutrition*, eds. Johnston I.D.A. and Lee H.A. *Research and Clinical Forums*, **1**, 35.

Chapter 2
Biochemical considerations

B. D. ROSS

The details of all the major metabolic pathways, and of some of the factors which regulate them, are known. Newer concepts, including the regulation of pathways by intermediates and metabolic products and by enzyme induction, are established, but our knowledge is incomplete. Classical biochemistry, derived from *in vitro* studies in experimental animals, has concentrated on the biochemistry of single organs, and only now is beginning to concern itself with the interactions between organs. These interactions may be of great importance in parenteral feeding. There is also objective evidence of the obvious clinical truth that sick patients differ from well individuals and from each other in their metabolism. Each individual undergoes a process of metabolic adaptation which may alter the relative rates of a number of alternative pathways of metabolism. Recent interest in parenteral feeding has been stimulated by the opportunities offered for legitimate metabolic studies in man and there has been an increasing interest in amino acid metabolism (see Felig, 1975, for review). In this chapter, some of the standard biochemical pathways will be reviewed and the following topics will be discussed:

The re-defining of the cause of negative nitrogen balance in trauma and surgical stress.

The recognition of metabolic heterogeneity in the patient's response to trauma and other clinical conditions.

The special role of branched-chain keto acids and branched-chain amino acids in protein synthesis.

The possibility that carnitine increases the utilisation of lipid in feeding regimens.

 B. D. Ross

Aims of parenteral feeding

The basic aim of parenteral nutrition is to maintain a good nutritional status in patients who cannot take food in adequate amounts either orally or enterally. The variety of clinical conditions covered by this simple aim is illustrated in Table 2.1. To this list may be added such problems as unhealed wounds, protein-losing enteropathy, diverticulitis, severe anorexia and so on. All these patients will be considered as a single problem, but different patterns of metabolic adaptation are beginning to emerge (see Chapter 6) and this may allow us to group them differently at some future date.

The 24-hour requirements for the maintenance of health in the 'average' adult have been extensively debated and constantly revised (American Medical Association, 1979). The immutable components are water, salt, fuels of respiration to provide ATP both for work and the maintenance of cellular integrity, specific amino acids for protein synthesis, 'essential' fatty acids, vitamins and co-factors, minerals and trace elements. There is no perfect regimen, and the painstaking collection of information on the minimum requirement of each trace

Table 2.1. *Indications for parenteral nutrition*

1. Preoperative conditions

2. Postoperative conditions

3. Post-traumatic conditions.   Burns

4. Malabsorption or when the gastrointestinal tract needs rest

short bowel syndrome	pancreatitis
severe enteritis	ulcerative colitis
peritonitis	Crohn's disease
ileus	gastrointestinal carcinoma

5. Fistulas

6. Unconsciousness when tube feeding is contraindicated

7. Other conditions with inadequate enteral feeding

chronic diarrhoea	cachexia
chronic vomiting	during radiation treatment
anorexia	treatment with cytostatic drugs

8. Premature infants

9. Kidney or liver insufficiency

(Modified from Wretlind, 1978)

element in well individuals is still going on. It is unlikely that our view of these requirements will change drastically.

The 14 or so commercially available amino acid mixtures are virtually interchangeable and are composed on a quite arbitrary basis. To avoid getting lost in detailed debate, the standard regimen which is issued by the Pharmacy of the John Radcliffe Hospital, Oxford, under the guidance of the Parenteral Nutrition Team, is shown in Table 2.2.

General biochemical considerations

The first step is to consider the major pathways of metabolism in order to rationalise the choice of a feeding regimen in detail. In the

Table 2.2. *Total parenteral nutrition. Standard formula used in the John Radcliffe Hospital, Oxford*

Carbohydrate (Glucose)	250 g
Nitrogen	14 g
Sodium	100 m mole
Potassium	100 m mole
Calcium	13 m mole
Magnesium	19 m mole
Phosphate	30 m mole
Zinc	0.24 m mole
Chloride	232 m mole
Folate	15 mg
Vitamins	
Thiamine	250 mg
Riboflavine	4 mg
Pyridoxine	50 mg
Nicotinamide	160 mg
Ascorbic Acid	500 mg
plus	
Fat Intralipid 20%	500 ml
All the above are given daily	
The following are given weekly	
Vitamins	
Vitamin A	75 mcg
Vitamin D	0.3 mcg
Vitamin K	15 mcg
Trace Elements	

final common pathway of energy metabolism, ATP is produced by
the activity of dehydrogenases and electron transport, the latter
occurring in mitochondria, which are found in virtually all cells, except
erythrocytes. The fate of ATP is conversion to creatine phosphate in
muscle (the high-energy compound of heart and skeletal muscle), or
hydrolysis, with the liberation of 10–11 kCals/mole ATP. Many
vitamins are immediate precursors of the co-factors participating in
substrate oxidation and the electron–transport chain and, as such,
are indispensable to life of the cell. (NAD = nicotinamide; CoA =
pantothenic acid; Flavoprotein = riboflavine; Iron–sulphate complex =
Fe^{++} and S''; TPP (of pyruvate dehydrogenase complex) = thiamin, and
so on).

Sources of energy

The energy required for metabolic processes is derived from three main
sources, namely, carbohydrates, amino acids and lipids.

The tricarboxylic acid cycle (TCA cycle) is the final common pathway of most cellular respiration, being the route of oxidation of 2–
carbon fragments (acetyl Coenzyme A) derived ultimately from glucose,
fatty acids and some amino acids. The cycle is under metabolic control,
and could conceivably be modified in sick patients; in fasting rats, the
maximum rate of the cycle is reduced by some 30–40% (Vinay *et al.*,
1978). But the TCA cycle is so central to life of the cell that great
variations in its individual reactions are not to be expected. Intermediates of the TCA cycle can be consumed by gluconeogenesis. Some
solutions offered for parenteral feeding contain malate, ostensibly to
'spark' oxidation of acetyl CoA. Its efficacy is uncertain and, anyway,
either glutamate or aspartate, which are included in most amino acid
mixtures, can readily form TCA intermediates, 2–oxoglutarate and
oxaloacetate respectively.

Carbohydrates

The most important carbohydrate is glucose. Formation of acetyl
CoA from carbohydrate follows the glycolytic pathway. The alternative pathway for glucose oxidation, the pentose phosphate shunt,
generates reducing co-factors required for fatty acid synthesis in the
anabolic cell. The importance of the pentose phosphate shunt in sick

patients, in whom fatty acid oxidation rather than synthesis is the order of the day, is quite unknown, and the attempt to exploit it by the use of xylitol as a carbon source has been disastrous.

Carbohydrates other than glucose have been used as an energy source in parenteral feeding. Given that insulin is essential for the optimum uptake of glucose by muscle and adipose tissue (but not by liver or brain), fructose or sorbitol might be seen as attractive alternatives, but both may give rise to severe lactic acidosis (Woods, 1974). Ethanol is another source of 2—carbon fragments for energy production; alcohol dehydrogenase, the first enzyme of the pathway, is in the liver. Serious metabolic derangements have accompanied its use (Cohen *et al.*, 1974).

Gluconeogenesis

Physicians employing parenteral nutrition should also be aware of gluconeogenesis, that is, glucose synthesis from non-carbohydrate sources. This is a major metabolic pathway, partly involving reversal of the reactions of glycolysis, whereby blood sugar levels are maintained. Lactate, formed by glycolysis in erythrocytes, alanine formed in muscle, and glycerol derived from lipolysis of triglycerides, are the major endogenous sources of glucose produced in this way. A major and usually undesirable fate of the carbon-chain of some amino acids is to form glucose. In starvation and in many ill patients, the adaptive increase of gluconeogenesis helps to maintain glucose levels; protein breakdown and the negative nitrogen balance are thus the expression of the overriding importance to the organism of the provision of glucose. Gluconeogenesis and its metabolic regulation have been the subject of innumerable *in vitro* studies. The rate of hepatic gluconeogenesis increases in prolonged fasting, due to the increased availability of substrates (proteolysis, glycolysis and lipolysis) and also due to enzyme induction. This increase in activity of the enzymes of gluconeogenesis in liver and kidney occurs under the influence of substrates and hormones.

Lipids

Lipids, the other major source of calories used in parenteral nutrition, are given largely as triglycerides, which are metabolised by lipolysis to glycerol (which is itself converted to glucose or oxidised by the glycoly-

B. D. Ross

tic pathway) and free fatty acids. The fatty acids may be completely oxidised, with the formation of considerable quantities of ATP, or be converted to ketone bodies, themselves now recognised as important fuels of respiration for brain and other tissues, or be converted back to triglycerides (Fig. 2.1). The conversion back to triglycerides is unlikely to occur to any great extent in seriously ill patients, in whom lipolysis predominates. The relative rates of fatty acid oxidation and ketone body production are under metabolic control. Ketosis may therefore be viewed either as a failure of metabolic regulation (as in diabetes) or as a means of providing an essential fuel for respiration under conditions in which other fuels are lacking.

In addition to calories, Intralipid provides the essential unsaturated fatty acids (linoleic, linolenic and arachidonic acids), in the absence of which deficiency diseases appear in patients receiving parenteral nutrition (McCarthy *et al.*, 1978). They are probably required for cell membrane synthesis and they are 'essential' in that they cannot be synthesised *de novo* in man.

Little work has been done on the alternative fuels of lipid origin which may be of value in parenteral nutrition. Medium chain triglycerides or short-chain fatty acids use different enzymes for activation during their oxidation; possibly there may be some advantages in this, but no work has been done with intravenous as opposed to orally administered medium chain triglycerides. Beta-hydroxybutyrate will be readily oxidised and restore nitrogen balance, at least in fasting man (Sherwin *et al.*, 1975). Glycerol-acetoacetate, another source of oxi-

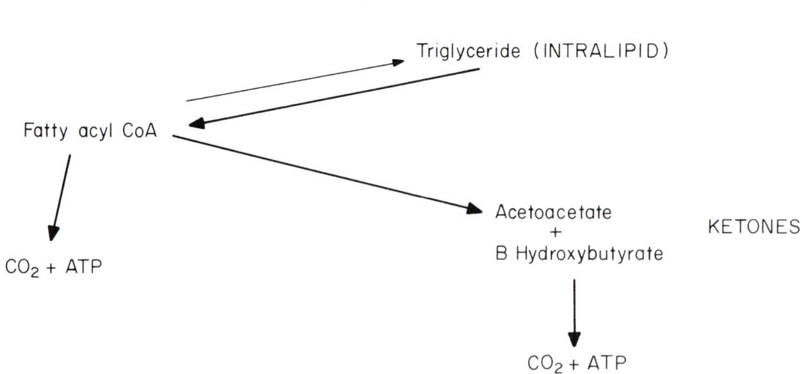

Fig. 2.1. *Fate of lipids.*

Table 2.3. *Comparison of carbohydrate and lipid as the source of calories in parenteral feeding*

Carbohydrate as calorie source

Advantages	*Disadvantages*
Readily assimilated	Irritant at high concentrations
Cheap 'nitrogen sparing'	Diuresis when renal threshold exceeded
Insulin promotes uptake	Insulin resistance of post-trauma patients
	Biochemical hazards of fuels other than glucose (fructose, sorbitol, xylitol)
	Lactacidosis
	Low energy yield 4 kcal/g

Lipid as calorie source

Advantages	*Disadvantages*
Small volume	Expensive
Non-irritant	? poorly utilised
'Essential' fatty acids provided	Ketogenic
Equal nitrogen sparing with carbohydrate	Unknown incidence of liver disease
High energy yield 9 kcal/g	No specific advantage over carbohydrate

Wretlind (1978), the originator of Intralipid, suggests that carbohydrate and lipid are of equal merit in the composition of parenteral feeding regimens.

dative fuel, which bypasses activation steps, has so far been tried only in rats (Birkhahn *et al.*, 1979). Intralipid itself has a somewhat poor reputation as it has been thought to be responsible for liver damage and all users are familiar with the persistent lipaemia which attends its use. However, it is difficult to find objective reports of adverse reactions to its use, and it is therefore legitimate to ask the question whether carbohydrate or lipid is to be preferred as a source of calories in parenteral feeding (Table 2.3).

Amino acids and nitrogen metabolism

Rightly or wrongly, the pervading view of parenteral feeding is that the maintenance of a positive nitrogen balance is the key to success. Nitrogen has been given in the form of amino acid mixtures of great variety, both in composition and cost. Our knowledge of the metabolic basis for the choice of amino acids is incomplete. The so-called 'essential' amino acids are phenylalanine, tryptophan, histidine, arginine, lysine, threonine and methionine, and the three branched-chain amino acids, valine, leucine and isoleucine. They are essential in that they cannot be synthesised by man and must be provided in any long-term feeding regimen. The role of arginine (or ornithine) as a catalyst in urea synthesis in liver will be recalled (Krebs and Henseleit, 1932). There is no objective evidence that ammonia accumulates in patients receiving parenteral feeding with amino acid mixtures not containing ornithine, but ornithine is included in all amino acid mixtures anyway.

Given that essential amino acids will continue to be included in parenteral feeding regimens until more information is available, what of non-essential amino acids? The metabolism of amino acids follows one of three general pathways: incorporation into protein with or without transamination; deamination, with conversion of the ammonia to urea and the carbon chain to either glucose or ketone bodies (amino acids are further classified as glucogenic or ketogenic); or complete oxidation to CO_2 with the formation of ATP. In terms of parenteral nutrition, only transamination is advantageous, since incorporation into protein can still follow; deamination and disposal of the carbon chain by whatever route must at present be viewed as a loss of vital ingredients of the regimen. For this reason, feeding regimens are at present designed to conserve infused amino acids and to minimise urea synthesis. Thus it is that the success of various procedures is judged by their ability to promote nitrogen retention. Nitrogen retention may be brought about by adding carbohydrate, lipid or insulin, or by increasing the rate of infusion of the amino acids (Table 2.4). In addition, branched-chain amino acids may have a special role over and above their 'essential' contribution.

Since fasting and some clinical conditions result in an adaptive increase in gluconeogenesis from amino acids, and since amino acids given alone act as an energy source if oxidised, the usual procedure is to administer an alternative source of calories at the same time as giving the amino acid mixture. The 'magic' figure of 200 kCal/g of amino acid is empirically derived and there is no very clear theoretical ideal. The earliest studies suggested that glucose was particularly effective in suppressing amino acid oxidation. Recent studies by Jeejeebhoy

Table 2.4. *Metabolic means of conserving amino acid nitrogen*

Substance	Effect
Alternative calorie supply	
Carbohydrate	inhibits ketogenesis
	inhibits gluconeogenesis
	conserves nitrogen
Fat	conserves nitrogen
Hormone effects	
Insulin	? inhibits gluconeogenesis
	promotes muscle amino acid uptake
	antagonises glucagon effect on liver
Anabolic steroids	?
Glucagon (lack of)	limits hepatic gluconeogenesis
Specific effectors of protein synthesis	
Leucine	in vitro, increase in amino acid uptake
	in vivo, disproportional effect on protein synthesis
Other branced chain amino acids	possibly the same effects
Branched chain keto-acids	effective in reducing nitrogen loss
	? mechanism as above

and his colleagues show sparing of amino acid nitrogen to be as effective with Intralipid as with glucose (Greenberg *et al.*, 1976).

Insulin can be expected to have an effect on the uptake of amino acids by muscle and it has recently been shown to have a measurable effect on nitrogen retention during parenteral nutrition of patients with burns (Woolfson *et al.*, 1979). The effect is distinct from any effect of calories, such as is seen when glucose is given, and has led to the view that insulin should be included in parenteral nutrition regimens. However, Munro (1979) has pointed out that insulin cannot be the only effector.

Once we have the essential amino acids, there is virtually no information as to which, if any, of the non-essential amino acids are necessary for successful nutrition. The bulk of amino acids in commercial solutions are 'non-essential', because such amino acids are cheap; their contribution to nitrogen balance or even their utilisation in man has not always been ascertained. Costs are often compared on the basis of pounds sterling per gram of nitrogen; but 'more' is not always 'best'. Experiments are required in man to show the utilisation and, more important, the precise fate of individual amino acids. In terms of protein synthesis, is glycine superior to glutamate, or is alanine superior to both of these? Royle has pioneered the approach of infusing single amino acids in control subjects and sick patients to determine their half life (Royle *et al.*, 1977; Elia *et al.*, 1980). In preliminary studies we have looked at the metabolic fate of glutamate, which is a favourite amino acid in some commercial mixtures, as it is very inexpensive. We find that the half life in control subjects and in sick patients is so short (about ten minutes) that individuals will easily cope with the amounts given during standard feeding regimens (Fig. 2.2). But, interestingly, we find clear indications that the metabolic fate of glutamate is different in sick patients than in controls. In brief, blood lactate levels fall during glutamate infusion in controls, but not in the sick; and, in the urine, aspartate appears in controls in greatly increased amounts but not in the sick patients ($p < 0.01$). In sick patients, urinary aspartate is replaced by glutamine, which is virtually absent in controls. Our present interpretation of these findings is that glutamate is removed from the blood at an equally high rate in control subjects and sick patients, but that its

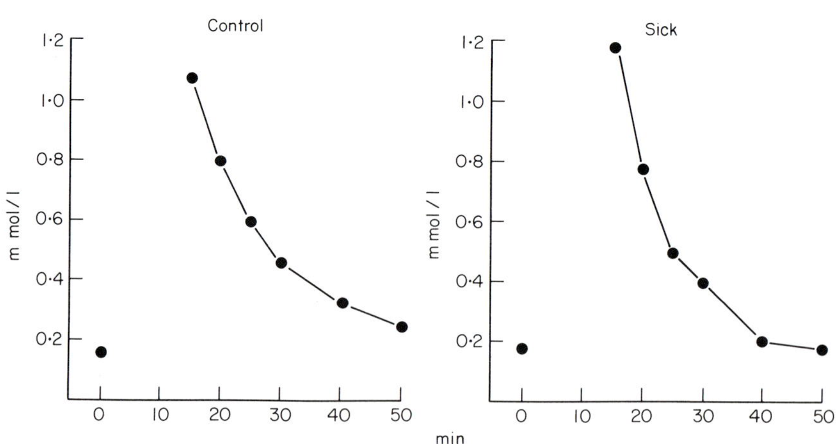

Fig. 2.2. *Removal of an intravenous load of Na-L-Glutamate in patients and controls.*

primary fate in controls is transamination (with nitrogen being conserved), while in the sick patients there may be impaired transamination,
so that some nitrogen derived from glutamate is lost. This observation
is in keeping with an early report that hepatic transaminase activity falls
rapidly in animals deprived of protein (Rosen *et al.*, 1959).

The hormonal regulation of metabolism in healthy man is reasonably
well understood and the molecular sites of action of the major hormones
are known. But the state of knowledge of the hormonal response to
severe disease and, further, of the modifications imposed by the feeding
of potent effectors of hormone release, such as glucose and amino acids,
is very confused. Measurement of circulating levels of hormones is not
necessarily helpful in these situations, in which cause and effect can
rarely be unravelled. A well controlled study by Woolfson *et al.* (1979)
confirms that the expected effect of insulin in promoting amino acid
uptake by skeletal muscle does indeed reverse negative nitrogen balance
during the parenteral feeding of patients with burns. But the interactions
with catecholamines, glucagon and glucocorticosteroids released (or
administered) in sick patients are unknown. Some amino acids themselves promote insulin release and part of the endocrine response
depends upon the gut (see below) so that intravenous amino acid
administration may complicate the picture still further (Fig. 2.3).

When nutrition is provided by the intravenous route, what are the
consequences to the patient of 'bypassing' the intestine in the metabolic sense? The answer is by no means clear but some effect is to be
anticipated. Windmueller and Spaeth (1974) have demonstrated that
important metabolic transformations take place in the gut wall after

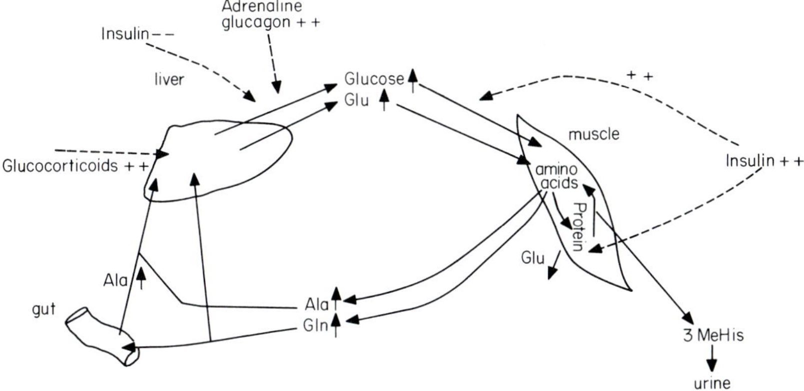

Fig. 2.3. *Hormonal and inter-organ influences on metabolism.*

normal feeding. Alanine is released and glutamine is formed from glutamate, so that glutamate will hardly ever reach the systemic circulation under normal dietary conditions. Since glutamate is a stimulant to insulin release, are we to expect a different response to intravenous glutamate given as a key ingredient of parenteral nutrition solutions (Cahill, 1972)? The gut is part of an important cycle of metabolic transformations carried out in conjunction with the liver, muscle and kidney, the full importance of which in the response to parenteral nutrition is still unclear.

Loss of the portal route of substrate delivery may limit transamination, glucose synthesis and urea synthesis. The release of insulin or inhibition of glucagon release which follows the delivery of high concentrations of amino acids in the portal circulation to the pancreas may have far-reaching effects on the metabolic response to disease. And the absence of the intestinal phase of digestion with the release of glucagon-like substances and other local hormones may be significant. We have no systematic information at present, but data will accumulate as more metabolic studies are undertaken in man in the search for better means of parenteral nutrition.

Specific developments which may influence future feeding regimens

The mechanism of the negative nitrogen balance

A negative nitrogen balance is not due to accelerated muscle breakdown in the majority of cases. This simple truth is perhaps the most important idea to enter the field of parenteral feeding in recent years, and it stems from the measurement of an unusual amino acid, 3-methyl histidine, in the urine. Although there have been a number of studies using other methods which pointed in the same direction (Smith *et al.*, 1975; Crane *et al.*, 1977), studies in Boston showed that muscle breakdown could be readily quantified by measuring 3-methyl histidine in the urine (Munro and Young, 1978). The histidine which is present in actin and in the heavy chain of myosin in fast muscle is methylated after the synthesis of actomyosin. After proteolysis, all amino acids except this methylated form are recycled for the synthesis of new protein. This problem has beset any investigation of the true rate of amino acid incorporation into protein. As 3-methyl histidine cannot be re-used and is excreted, in constitutes a quantitative marker of the mass of protein which has been broken down. Thus, fracture of a long bone in a rat produces an increased nitrogen loss, but no change in 3-methyl histidine excretion, so that it is failure of protein synthesis and not increased protein breakdown which causes the excessive nitrogen loss. The consequences of this finding for parenteral nutrition remain to be fully explored: we need to find agents which will remove the block to protein synthesis; pouring in amino acids without removing the block may eventually prove to have been an expensive waste.

The role of branched-chain amino acids in protein synthesis

A clue came from observations on isolated muscle. Leucine, one of the essential branched-chain amino acids, appears to play a disproportionate role in stimulating amino acid uptake and *de novo* protein synthesis (Odessy and Goldberg, 1972). In man, the branched-chain keto-acids (analogues of the amino acids), which are used in the management of some forms of uraemia, reverse the negative nitrogen balance of starvation (Sapir and Walser, 1977). It is therefore likely that the carbon chain is important for protein synthesis. Freund *et al.* (1979) found that an infusion containing only branched-chain amino acids was as effective as a full mixture of amino acids in reversing the nitrogen excretion of mild surgical trauma. As we now know, this represents the promotion of protein synthesis and not the reversal of muscle breakdown. It remains to be seen whether this special effect will be of practical value in parenteral nutrition. It is, after all, anomalous that it is just the branched-chain amino acids which accumulate in the blood after trauma (Wedge *et al.*, 1976). Why are they unable to stimulate protein synthesis under these conditions?

Metabolic heterogeneity in the response to trauma and disease

Both the need for parenteral nutrition and the likely course of the response to it are dictated by the metabolic adaptation in man which occurs in response to the insult of disease. The best-understood adaptation is that to fasting, which in animals increases the rate of hepatic and renal gluconeogenesis, and of hepatic ketogenesis and urea synthesis, within a few hours. The most detailed studies in man have been extended to six weeks of starvation and have demonstrated a sequence of metabolic adaptations (Owen and Cahill, 1973). The responses to administered intravenous fuels in patients at different stages of this adaptation are likely to be different, although this has not been properly studied. The adaptation to trauma can follow two distinct patterns: ketotic and non-ketotic. The patients who fall into the non-ketotic group appear to suffer the more severe metabolic damage, with increased nitrogen excretion, increased circulating branched-chain amino acids, and increased excretion of 3-methyl histidine (Smith *et al.*, 1975; Wedge *et al.*, 1976; Williamson *et al.*, 1977).

On this basis, it would indeed be surprising if patients did not respond differently to parenteral nutrition depending upon the nature of their primary response to trauma. We must conclude that we are looking at a heterogeneous population (Munro, 1979). This is not by any means a new idea to the clinician, but the final classification may not resemble anything that we are currently using and may profoundly influence the type of parenteral nutrition regimens in the future.

Limitations upon the rate of utilisation of nutritional lipid

There is a possible way by which the usefulness of Intralipid might be extended. A closer look at the pathway of fatty acid oxidation and ketone body synthesis reveals an absolute requirement for the triamino-acid, carnitine (Fig. 2.4). Carnitine is not a vitamin, since it is probably formed in sufficient quantities from 3-aminobutyric acid in muscle. Its urinary excretion is greatly increased after trauma (Maebashi *et al.*, 1977). The infusion of Intralipid does not significantly depress blood levels of carnitine, but does halve its urinary excretion (König *et al.*, 1978).

It is tempting to suggest that the relatively slow rate of removal of Intralipid from blood (as shown by the lipaemic serum in many patients receiving it) may be a limitation set by the amount of carnitine available to cope with the excessive load of lipid. Our preliminary studies lend a little support to this idea but are by no means conclusive. When two infusions of Intralipid were given in sequence, allowing one day for 'recovery', the rise in plasma triglyceride was accompanied by ketone body formation, and both fell to normal again within a few hours,

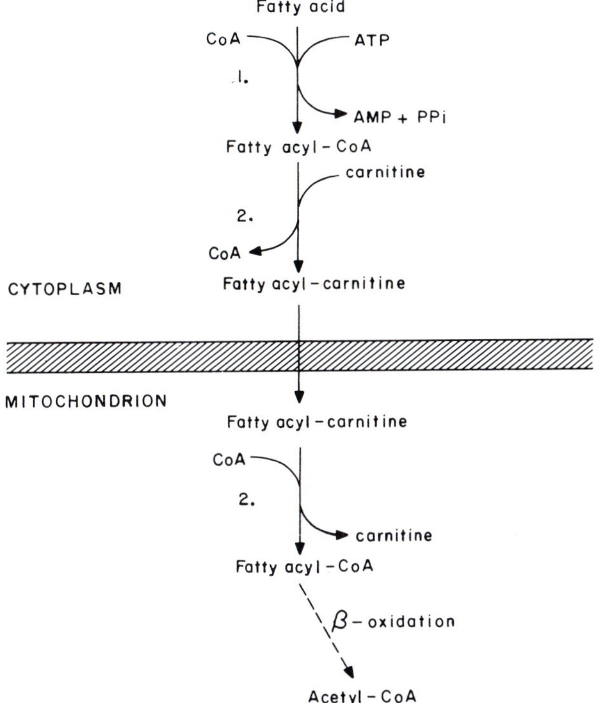

Fig. 2.4. *Role of carnitine in fatty acid oxidation (modified from Newsholme and Start, 1973).*

before the second Intralipid infusion. The elevation in serum trigly-cerides was nevertheless very significantly greater in response to this second load, while ketone body formation was significantly less. This means that there was impairment of lipid oxidation. We know too that carnitine excretion was greatly diminished during and following the first Intralipid infusion. Giving supplementary D–L carnitine by mouth with either the first or the second lipid infusion had no effect on the maximum level of serum triglyceride achieved. But an effect was noted on ketone body formation. In response to the second lipid infusion, ketone body formation was much more nearly normal in patients receiving carnitine than in those who did not. This preliminary evidence of a role for carnitine must be treated cautiously but, if substantiated, may justify the inclusion of carnitine in parenteral nutrition regimens to enhance the utilisation of intravenous lipids. In principle, the idea of co-factor limitation in the face of very high intravenous loads may be extended to other agents and substrates.

Conclusions

The aim of parenteral feeding is to provide the nutritional requirements for metabolism and thus aid recovery from severe trauma or disease. An understanding of the general metabolic pathways allows a standard regimen to be designed to meet most requirements.

In the future, it will be important to distinguish between patients with increased muscle breakdown and those with impaired protein synthesis. Furthermore, it will be necessary to recognise different patterns of response to trauma or systemic disease, for example, ketotic or non-ketotic. Branched-chain amino acids, insulin and carnitine may each prove to have a specific role in parenteral feeding.

In principle, the regimen of parenteral nutrition should be designed to take account of individual requirements.

ACKNOWLEDGEMENTS

I am grateful to my colleagues, Miss Penelope Kingsland, Mrs Sylvia Bartlett, Dr Peter Rawcliffe and Mr Andrew Kingsnorth for allowing me to mention some of our joint unpublished work. Miss Penelope Kingsland has been supported by Travenol (UK) Ltd., and Mrs Sylvia Bartlett by a grant from the Oxfordshire Area Health Authority.

References

American Medical Association, Department of Food and Nutrition (1979) *J. Amer. med. Ass.* **241**, 2051.

Birkhahn R.H., McMenamy R.H. and Border J.R. (1979) *J. Nutr.* **109**, 1168.

Cahill G.H. (1972) Discussion remark in *Intravenous Hyperalimentation,* eds. Cowan G.S.M. and Scheetz W.L., Lea and Febriger, Philadelphia, p. 52.

Cohen R.D., Woods H.F. and Alberti K.G. (1974) *Lancet,* i, 405.

Crane C.W., Picou D., Smith R. and Waterlow J.C. (1977) *Brit. J. Surg.* **64**, 129.

Elia M., Ilic V., Bacon S., Williamson D.H. and Smith R. (1980) *Clin. Sci.* (in press).

Felig P. (1975) *Ann. Rev. Biochem.* **44**, 933.

Freund H., Hoover H.C., Atamain S. and Fischer J.E. (1979) *Ann. Surg.* **190**, 18.

Greenberg G.R., Marliss E.B., Anderson G.H., Langer B., Spence W., Toree E.B. and Jeejeebhoy K.N. (1976) *New Engl. J. Med.* **294**, 1411.

Jeejeebhoy K.N., Langez B., Tsallis G. *et al.* (1976) *Gastroenterology,* **76**, 943.

Konig B., McCaigney E., Conteh S. and Ross B.D. (1978) *Clin. Chem Acta,* **88**, 121.

Krebs H.A. and Henseleit K. (1932) *Ztsch. f. physiol. chem.* **210**, 33.

Maebashi M., Kawmura N., Sato M. *et al.* (1977) *Metabolism,* **26**, 357.

McCarthy D.M., May R.J., Maher M. and Brennan M.K. (1978) *Am. J. Dig. Dis.* **23**, 1009.

Munro H.N. (1979) *New Engl. J. Med.* **300**, 41.

Newsholme E.A. and Start C. (1973) *Regulation in Metabolism,* Wiley, London.

Odessey R. and Goldberg A.L. (1972) *Amer. J. Physiol.* **223**, 1376.

Owen O.E. and Cahill G.F. (1973) *J. clin. Invest.* **52**, 2596.

Rosen F., Roberts N.R. and Nichol C.A. (1959) *J. biol. Chem.* **234**, 476.

Royle G., Kettlewell M., Ilic V. and Williamson D.H. (1978) *Brit. J. Surg.* **65**, 363.

Sapir D.G. and Walser M. (1977) *Metabolism,* **26**, 301.

Sherwin R.S., Hendler R.G. and Felig P. (1975) *J. clin. Invest.* **55**, 1382.

Smith R., Fuller D.J., Wedge J.H., Williamson D.H. and Alberti K.G.G.M. (1975) *Lancet,* i, 1.

Vinay P., Mapes J.P. and Krebs H.A. (1978) *Amer. J. Physiol.* **234**, F123.

Wedge J.H., DeCampos R., Kerr A., Smith R., Farrell R., Ilic V. and Williamson D.H. (1976) *Clin. Sci. Mol. Med.* **50**, 393.

Williamson D.H., Farrell R., Kerr A. and Smith R. (1977) *Clin. Sci. Mol. Med.* **52**, 527.

Windmueller H.G. and Spaeth A.E. (1974) *J. biol. Chem.* **249**, 5070.

Woods H.F. (1974). In *Topics in Gastroenterology 2,* ed. Truelove S.C. and Trowell J., p. 191. Blackwell Scientific Publications.

Woolfson A.J., Heatley R.V. and Allison S.P. (1979) *New Engl. J. Med.* **300**, 14.

Wretlind A. (1978) *Surg. Clin. N. Amer.* **58**, 1055.

Young V.R. and Munro H.N. (1978) *Fed. Proc.* **37**, 2291.

Chapter 3
Practical aspects

M. G. W. KETTLEWELL

Parenteral nutrition is widely accepted as a powerful therapeutic tool, but it is potentially hazardous, and over-enthusiastic use in many countries has produced a rich harvest of complications, some of which have been fatal. Many hospitals in the United States of America include in their hospital manual several pages of the complications of parenteral nutrition. It has been shown repeatedly that close attention to the practical details of parenteral nutrition should minimize the complications, both in number and severity (Bernard and Stahl, 1971; Ellis *et al.*, 1976).

Parenteral nutrition team

A small group or team is the core of successful parenteral nutrition in any hospital big enough to use this form of nutritional support regularly (Ryan, 1976). The team should contain at least a clinician, a nurse and a pharmacist, and, ideally, a biochemist and a dietician as well. The members of the team, with diverse expertise but a common interest, stimulate ideas and arrive at solutions to particular problems, as well as ensuring a high standard of sympathetic care. The team should be able to function across traditional clinical barriers and should offer a service rather than attempting to take over the entire management of the patient.

Selection of patients

Parenteral nutrition is not a nutritional panacea, and therefore careful selection of patients for this form of therapy is the first practical problem that faces the team. The indications for TPN are dealt with more fully in Chapter 4. Nutritional support of hospital patients should be considered early, and the alternatives to parenteral nutrition should be employed whenever feasible. TPN should be reserved for those patients who cannot, or should not, use the gastro-intestinal tract.

Method of delivery

Most parenteral nutrition solutions are hyperosmolar and acidic compared to blood or plasma, and they irritate the venous endothelium sufficiently to cause thrombo-phlebitis, particularly in the smaller peripheral veins which are used for most infusions. The choice of access to the circulation for the infusion of nutrients therefore lies between using a central or peripheral vein. This choice is governed by the requirements of the patient and the resulting choice of nutrient solutions. For example, it is reasonable to use peripheral veins post-operatively in previously healthy patients when a prolonged post-operative course is expected. If peripheral veins are used, then the infusion site needs to be changed every 24—48 hours, and the osmolality of the infusate reduced by lowering the calorie input and using intralipid for approximately half the calories. This method of parenteral nutrition is widely practised in Sweden (Grotte *et al.*, 1976).

Central veins are used in most patients who depend on parenteral nutrition to survive because of their need for high concentrations of glucose as a major energy source. These patients seldom have adequate peripheral veins for continuous use, and in practised hands the central vein is a safe and comfortable access site. Although there are various means of access to the superior vena cava (Table 3.1), infraclavicular subclavian vein puncture is the most widely practised. It is as easy to

Table 3.1. *Central vein access sites*

1. Long antecubital vein catheter.
2. Internal jugular vein puncture.
3. External jugular vein puncture.
4. Supraclavicular subclavian puncture.
5. Infraclavicular subclavian puncture.

perform as the other methods, and once in place the catheter is more comfortable for the patient and easier to look after than when the jugular or supraclavicular approaches are employed. The long ante-cubital vein catheter is uncomfortable for the patient and is liable to become infected because of movement of the elbow; it may also provoke an axillary vein thrombosis. The common femoral vein is a potentially dangerous site, because of the increased risk of ilio-femoral vein thrombosis and catheter-induced septicaemia from the groin. The techniques of insertion of central vein catheters are well described by Karran and Norman (1980) but it is a matter for debate whether feeding lines should only be inserted in an operating theatre. Providing the clinician inserting the line maintains a thorough aseptic technique, there is, in my opinion, little advantage to be gained by using an operating theatre rather than a ward side-room.

The choice of central catheter is of considerable importance, since stiff catheters may injure the superior vena cava, and poor manufac-ture may lead to cracked lower hubs which are associated with increased line infection (personal observation). It is our practice to use a Vygon silastic catheter inserted below the clavicle and tunnelled onto the anterior chest wall (Powell-Tuck, 1980; Mitchell *et al.*, 1980). There is some evidence that a tunnelled catheter reduces the skin-borne line infections (Broviac and Scribner, 1974).

Prevention of sepsis

Catheter-related sepsis is the most serious and persistent practical problem in Total Parenteral Nutrition. The alarming frequency of infection in the early days of parenteral nutrition casts doubt on the use of this form of treatment, but the evolution of parenteral nutrition teams and attention to detail has reduced line infection to 5% or less (Ryan, 1976).

Aseptic insertion of feeding lines and the use of buried silastic catheters are important, but the day-to-day care of the lines is crucial in preventing infection. There are no controlled studies that provide data on the best means of dressing feeding catheters, the frequency of dressing changes, or the frequency of changes of the giving set. How-ever, remarkably similar practical methods of managing lines have evolved independently in many centres. Firstly, the feeding lines are used only for feeding and for nothing else. This precludes the use of feeding lines for the giving of drugs, for blood-transfusion or for taking blood samples. The continuity of the infusion line is interrupted as infrequently as possible because the risk of introducing infection is increased each time the line is interrupted to change a bottle or a giving set. The 3-litre infusion bags are much better than multiple bottles as the infusion set is then changed only once a day (Mitchell *et al.*, 1980).

The puncture site needs to be cleaned and dressed at intervals using aseptic techniques, in order to prevent the accumulation of serum or sweat and skin bacteria around the catheter entry site. It appears that daily changes of dressing are unnecessarily frequent, and it is preferable to change the dressings every 48 hours.

If a patient becomes pyrexial while receiving parenteral nutrition, it is necessary to examine clinically and bacteriologically all other possible sites of infection before incriminating the central vein catheter. Blood samples should be taken immediately for culture and it is then reasonable to treat the patient with an antibiotic effective against most skin organisms. If the temperature fails to settle in 24–48 hours, the catheter should be withdrawn and the tip cultured. If the central venous catheter is the source of infection, the patient will respond rapidly to antibiotic treatment and withdrawal of the catheter. A new catheter may then be inserted after a delay of twenty-four hours. Alternatively the catheter may be changed over a guide wire using the Seldinger technique.

Choice of parenteral nutrition solutions

The choice of parenteral nutrition solutions for individual patients is often difficult, and this difficulty is compounded by the array of mixtures available commercially. The lack of firm metabolic data derived from the majority of patients requiring parenteral nutrition, who are septic and semi-starved, means that there are no firm guide lines. The majority of metabolic studies have been performed either on patients after uncomplicated elective operations or on patients critically ill after major injury or severe burns. Although such studies are of great importance, they have little practical value when feeding patients with, for example, a small bowel fistula or severe Crohn's disease.

Starting from first principles, parenteral nutrition solutions should mimic, as far as is practicable, the normal food intake, with comparable proportions of amino-nitrogen, carbohydrates, fat, minerals and vitamins. These need only be varied for known metabolic disturbances, such as occur after severe burns or with liver failure. We have found that 75% of our patients requiring parenteral nutrition are managed simply and successfully on a standard nutrition regimen (Table 3.2), with only minor modifications of electrolyte content (Royle *et al.*, 1980). The remaining patients are catabolic or have severe liver or pulmonary disease, and these require substantial modification of nutrients.

Carbohydrate has been the main energy source but the provision of sufficient calories from glucose has often produced problems with glycosuria and hyperglycaemia. In particular, with hypercatabolic patients, who require substantial carbohydrate calories, large doses of exogenous insulin may be needed to maintain normoglycaemia (Woolfson, 1980). In the majority of patients it is simpler and safer to provide half the calories as glucose and half as fat (Intralipid). In these circumstances hyperglycaemia is seldom seen (Royle *et al.*, 1980).

Poor glucose utilization after injury has led to the use of fructose, sorbitol and xylitol, which are rapidly cleared from the blood and are not associated with hyperglycaemia. The disadvantages of these solutions, however, far outweigh their benefits, and seldom, if ever, is their use justified (Woods, 1974).

Most commercially available synthetic amino acid solutions have theoretically satisfactory biochemical profiles and are virtually indistinguishable. Most of them contain large quantities of either the glucogenic amino acids, alanine and glutamate, or the inexpensive amino acid,

Table 3.2. *The Oxford standard parenteral nutrition regimen*

Carbohydrate	250 g	
Nitrogen	14 g	
Sodium	100 m.mol	
Potassium	100 m.mol	
Calcium	13 m.mol	
Magnesium	19 m.mol	in 2·5 litres
Zinc	0.24 m.mol	
Phosphate	30 m.mol	
Multivitamins	10 ml	
Folic acid	15 mg	
Intralipid 20%	500 ml	

glycine. There is no clear evidence to favour or incriminate any of these amino acids. Whichever solution is used, most workers advocate that the nitrogen : calorie ratio should be approximately 1 : 150 (Kinney, 1980).

Some workers have suggested that the nutritional requirements of individual patients need to be tailored on a daily basis using numerous anthropometric and metabolic parameters. This requires sophisticated monitoring and the use of bedside computers. In Oxford, we have elected to use the simplest approach possible, which means that we give a standard solution to the majority of patients, and only tailor the regimen for the few critically ill patients (Royle *et al.*, 1980).

The addition of the minerals magnesium, zinc, and phosphate, as well as the complete range of vitamins, including folic acid, to feeding mixtures is now standard practice, but is easily forgotten. Trace elements and Vitamin B_{12} are only required for those patients supported intravenously for several weeks or months.

Delivery of parenteral nutrient solutions

The method of delivery of nutrient solutions to the patient is an important practical problem and depends to a large extent on the solution chosen. The simplest and most flexible method is to use the 3-litre bags filled with all the nutrients to be infused over 24 hours. The simplicity lies in the fact that a full day's requirements are delivered to the ward in one container, and the feeding line is interrupted only once each day. Greater flexibility can also be achieved using the larger bags rather than the commercially available 500 ml bottles, since the amounts of compatible solutions and electrolytes added to the bag can be varied almost at will. To achieve comparable flexibility using bottles, a vast range of infrequently used solutions would have to be stocked in the pharmacy. Substantial savings are also possible if 3-litre bags are used, and bulk purchases made of relatively few commercial solutions. Our pharmacy only stocks Synthamin 14 and 17 (Travenol), electrolyte solution A (Travenol), glucose 50% (Travenol) and Intralipid (Kabi-Vitrum) in addition to the other commonly available electrolyte solutions, vitamins and some trace element solutions. Nutrients from the 3-litre bag are delivered evenly and pre-mixed into the circulation with the exception of Intralipid, which is infused though a Y connection, in much the same way as nutrients are absorbed from the intestine, whereas nutrients in separate bottles, even when delivered through a Y or W drip set connection, tend to be delivered unevenly.

Filled 3-litre bags can be kept safely in a 4°C fridge for at least 48 hours. This allows parenteral feeds to be made up 24–48 hours in advance, and caters for pharmacy staffing difficulties at weekends. The use of 3-litre bags, however, requires tireless cooperation from the hospital pharmacy, since the solution, bags and giving sets must be handled aseptically in a clean environment and the bags filled under a laminar flow hood (Giovanni, 1976). It is also vitally important that the pharmacist has a sound knowledge of the compatibility of nutrient solutions. Once the bag has been filled, the drip set is attached aseptically and the whole assembly delivered to the ward.

Control of infusion

Intravenous infusions are notorious for becoming disconnected, running too fast or too slow, or becoming clotted because the drip has been turned off before changing the bottle. These problems, which are a nuisance with peripheral fluid infusions, are positively dangerous with central lines and parenteral nutrition. A regular infusion of nutrients over 24 hours is important and, if the 3-litre bag is used, it is also important to avoid accidental rapid infusion of all 3 litres. The ordinary resistance device on most giving sets is too unreliable for safe use. Many people have therefore used infusion pumps, which are either regulated by drop counters or are volumetrically controlled. Both types of pump have built-in safety devices to prevent infusion of air. These pumps are satisfactory and reliable for parenteral nutrition, but they are expensive and the volumetric pumps require special and fairly expensive giving sets with pumping cassettes. An alternative is to use a 'Dial-a-Flo' resistance device (Sorenson Ltd). (Fig. 3.1) This variable fluid resistance is attached by the pharmacist to the 3-litre bag grip set. The Intralipid line is inserted into the side-arm distal to the resistance (Mitchell *et al.*, 1980). The rate of infusion varies with the viscosity of the fluid, but the relationship between dial setting and flow rate remains linear. (Fig. 3.2) The infusion rate is also altered in an almost linear manner by the height of the infusion above the patient. Intralipid infusion through the side-arm, however, has no effect on the performance of the Dial-a-Flo (Mitchell *et al.*, 1980). We have used this device for over 1,500 patient-days, and have found it to be practical, safe, reliable and economical for the control of parenteral nutrition.

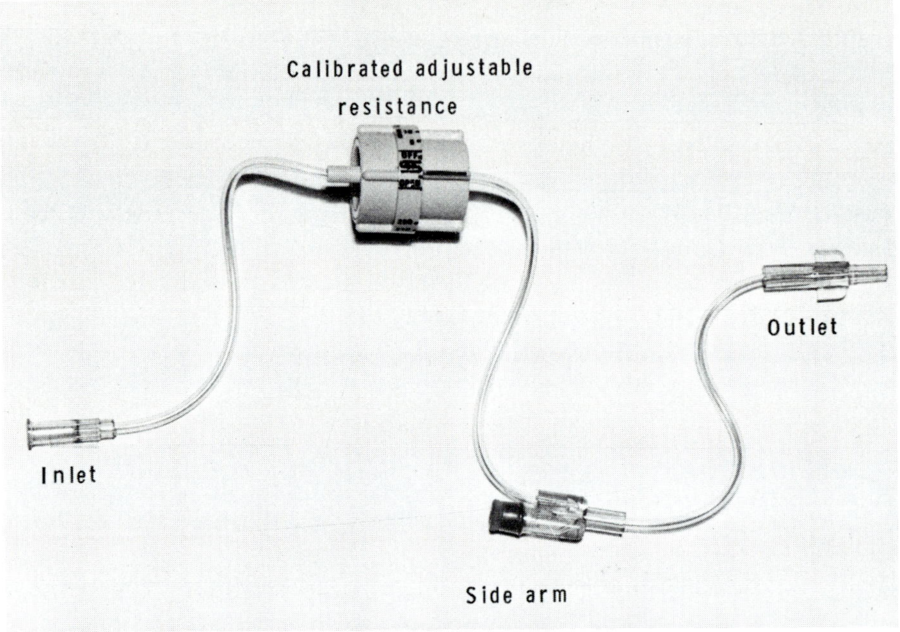

Fig. 3.1. *Dial-a-Flo (Sorenson Ltd). A resistance device for controlling the rate of infusion from a 3-litre bag.*

Monitoring the metabolic effect of TPN

Metabolic considerations and the risk of complications demonstrate the importance of monitoring the effect of parenteral nutrition. The variables that need to be monitored depend on how ill the patient is. For example, in patients who are severely ill and are being fed parenterally, their blood and urine electrolytes, nitrogen balance, plasma phosphate, magnesium and glucose, as well as haematological and liver function tests, need to be performed frequently, possibly daily, for the first few days of feeding. This intensive monitoring is necessary because critically ill patients are unable to handle excesses or deficiencies of nutrients as effectively as subjects who are merely malnourished. Malnourished patients, who have, for instance, dysphagia, and who are being prepared with parenteral nutrition for elective surgery, require less frequent monitoring. Biochemical and haematological studies should be done at least twice in the first week, but thereafter it is sufficient to repeat them weekly. It is important in all patients to

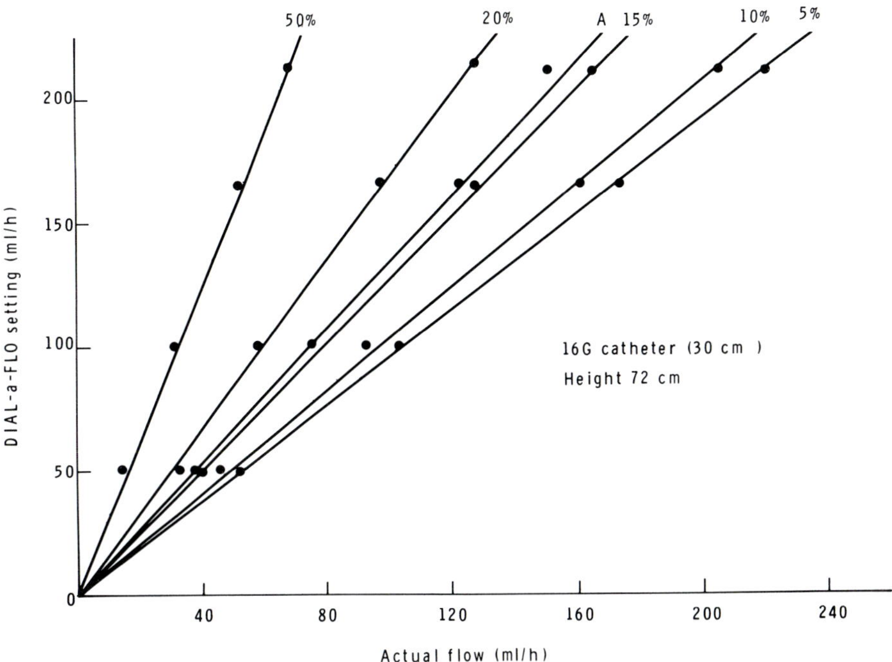

Fig. 3.2. *The relationship between Dial-a-Flo setting, viscosity and actual drip rate.*

measure nitrogen balance frequently as an index of the efficacy of parenteral nutrition (Lee, 1980).

Since sepsis is the single most important hazard it is important to perform blood culture at least weekly and whenever the patient is pyrexial.

Financial aspects

Parenteral nutrition is expensive, and it is clearly the nutrition team's duty to minimize the cost of this form of treatment, whether it is borne by the patient or by the State. Firstly, parenteral nutrition should only be used when absolutely necessary, rather than as a matter of routine. The choice, preparation and delivery of the nutrient solution should be governed not only by convenience and safety, but also by economic necessity. All reasonable means of economizing should be taken in relation to the methods of control of infusion and the type of delivery system used. At the time of writing, the cost of parenteral nutrition is about £50.00 per day per patient, and this fact should be considered before prescribing TPN.

ACKNOWLEDGEMENT

Fig. 3.2 is reproduced by permission of the Editors of the Annals of the Royal College of Surgeons of England.

References

Bernard R.W. and Stahl W.M. (1971) *Ann. Surg.* **173**, 184.

Broviac J.W. and Scribner B.H. (1974) *Surg. Gynec. Obst.* **139**, 24.

Ellis B.W., Stanbridge R. de L., Fielding L.P. and Dudley H.A.F. (1976) *Brit. med. J.* i, 1388.

Giovanni R. (1976). In *Total Parenteral Nutrition,* ed. Fischer J.E. Little, Brown, Boston.

Grotte G., Jacobson S. and Wretlind A. (1976). In *Total Parenteral Nutrition,* ed. Fischer J.E., Little, Brown, Boston.

Karran S.J. and Norman J. (1980). In *Practical Nutritional Support,* ed. Karran S.J. and Alberti K.G.M.M. Pittman Medical, Tunbridge Wells.

Kinney J.M. (1980). In *Practical Nutritional Support,* ed. Karran S.J. and Alberti K.G.M.M. Pittman Medical, Tunbridge Wells.

Lee H.A. (1980). In *Practical Nutritional Support,* ed. Karran S.J. and Alberti K.G.M.M. Pittman Medical, Tunbridge Wells.

Mitchell A., Draper C., Lee D.R., Royle G.T. and Kettlewell M.G.W. (1980) *Ann. Roy. Coll. Surg. Engl.* In press.

Powell, Tuck J. (1980). In *Practical Nutritional Support,* ed. Karran S.J. and Alberti K.G.M.M. Pittman Medical, Tunbridge Wells.

Royle G.T., Lee D.R., Draper C. and Kettlewell M.G.W. (1980) Awaiting publication.

Ryan I.A. (1976). In *Total Parenteral Nutrition,* ed. Fischer J.E. Little, Brown, Boston.

Woods H.F. (1974). In *Topics in Gastroenterology* 2, ed. Truelove S.C. and Trowell J. Blackwell Scientific Publications, Oxford.

Woolfson A.M.W. (1980). In *Practical Nutritional Support.* ed. Karran S.J. and Alberti K.G.M.M. Pittman Medical, Tunbridge Wells.

Chapter 4
Indications and contraindications

GRAHAM L. HILL

In patients in whom the gastrointestinal tract is blocked, too short, or extensively inflamed, parenteral nutrition may be required to maintain nutritional integrity. Some other very ill patients, in spite of an anatomically normal gastrointestinal tract, cannot ingest or absorb sufficient nutrients to maintain protein and energy balance, and parenteral feeding may be required in them also.

Intravenous nutrition (IVN) is now established as a safe and effective treatment for patients with a wide variety of clinical conditions. Although the value of IVN is seen most dramatically in newborns suffering from catastrophic gastrointestinal anomalies (Dudrick *et al.*, 1969), its use in adult patients with certain types of alimentary failure (Jacobson, 1972; Macfadyen *et al.*, 1973) and hypercatabolic illness (Liljedahl, 1972) has unquestionably led to decreased morbidity and mortality. It is now possible to feed patients entirely by the intravenous route for months or even years (Broviac *et al.*, 1973; Jeejeebhoy *et al.*, 1976; Solassol *et al.*, 1974) and most large hospitals have the skills and equipment to administer this treatment safely and effectively to any patient in whom it is strongly indicated. The treatment itself, however, is not without its dangers and in many patients alternative methods of nutritional therapy may be given more easily and they can be just as effective (Yeung *et al.*, 1979).

Indications for intravenous nutrition

It is not always easy to decide when and to whom IVN should be given. In the broadest terms it might be said that IVN should be considered whenever the gastrointestinal tract is *blocked, too short, inflamed* or simply *cannot cope.*

Applications of IVN when the gastrointestinal tract is blocked

Although acute obstruction of the small or large intestine is usually treated as a surgical emergency, any condition that gradually produces obstruction of the pharynx, oesophagus, stomach or duodenum may first require IVN to treat the insidious and often advanced malnutrition that has occurred. It is argued that malnutrition associated with profound weight loss (Studley, 1936), hypoproteinemia (Cannon *et al.*, 1944) and immune incompetence (Meakins *et al.*, 1977) is an adverse prognostic factor and materially affects the outcome of the major operation that may be required to relieve the obstruction. Available evidence suggests that weight loss must be very large (probably more than 20%), protein reserves must be severely depleted (about 20% or more of total body protein) and plasma protein concentrations very low (plasma albumin <30 g/l; plasma transferrin <150 mg %) before there is unequivocal statistical evidence that the outcome after surgery will be affected (Hill, 1979; Mullen *et al.*, 1979). Although patients with less severe malnutrition may not have an enhanced risk of developing a major surgical complication, should one occur they may be unable to withstand the subsequent nutritional assault. Thus, although patients with weight loss of more than 20%, and those with very low concentrations of plasma proteins should be fed intravenously for at least 2 weeks before a major operation, others, who on physical examination have depleted reserves of protein and fat, yet do not fulfil these criteria, should be considered carefully for pre-operative IVN. This is particularly so if it is considered that the post-operative course may be complicated. Malnourished patients requiring a major oesophageal or upper gastric resection should always be considered for pre-operative IVN, although it must be realised that this form of treatment can be associated with complications of its own. For example, in a recent study, an increased incidence of deep venous thrombosis was noted in patients treated in this way (Heatley *et al.*, 1976).

Applications of IVN when the gastrointestinal tract is too short

After massive resection of the small intestine, the patient is unable to maintain nutritional integrity by the oral route for weeks or months. In some patients, this is never achieved and parenteral nutrition is required indefinitely. More often, however, parenteral nutrition will be required for 6—8 weeks after which time sufficient adaptation (i.e. a stool loss of less than 2 litres in 24 hours) will have occurred to allow the cautious administration of a formula-defined diet. These diets are devoid of, or are low in, long-chain fatty acids and contain a mixture of essential amino acids, glucose, balanced electrolytes and other nutrients (Young *et al.*, 1975).

It is important that the transition to oral feeding be gradual and completion of the process may take several months, depending on the length, condition and degree of adaptation of the remaining small intestine. Parenteral nutrition should not be stopped until it is apparent that the patient can sustain his nutrition by the oral route.

For patients in whom adequate adaptation does not occur, long-term parenteral nutrition at home will be required. An indwelling silastic catheter is placed in the superior vena cava of the patient and nutrient solutions, mixed at home, are infused each day. This is usually carried out at night so permitting near-normal activities during the day (Fleming *et al.*, 1977; Ladefoged and Jarnum, 1978). Home parenteral nutrition is an important development in the treatment of patients with the short gut syndrome who cannot be maintained by oral feeding.

High output external small bowel fistulas, with losses of more than 500 ml of fluid per 24 hours, are best treated with total parenteral nutrition. Once sepsis is controlled and such treatment is instituted, it can be expected that 60—70% of such fistulas will close without the need for surgical intervention (Blackett and Hill, 1978; Macfadyen *et al.*, 1973). There is evidence that maintenance of an adequate nutritional state has lowered the mortality of this condition (Leading Article, *Lancet,* 1979) but parenteral nutrition is also probably associated with decreased output of fluid, electrolytes and enzymes (Towne *et al.*, 1973) and this presumably promotes healing of the fistula.

Applications of IVN when the gastrointestinal tract is inflamed

Nutritional depletion is a common feature of inflammatory bowel disease. More than 50% of patients requiring urgent surgery for acute colitis, for instance, suffer from protein calorie malnutrition of a degree which could interfere with immunocompetence, wound healing and rehabilitation after surgery (Hill *et al.*, 1977). Such patients may benefit from a post-operative course of parenteral nutrition and there is some evidence that this can be beneficial (Collins *et al.*, 1978).

It is much more difficult to decide if a regimen of bowel rest and total parenteral nutrition is of primary therapeutic help in patients with inflammatory bowel disease.

There are reports of patients who had not responded to the usual medical measures going into remission when the gut was rested and vigorous nutritional therapy instituted (Driscoll and Rosenberg, 1978). There is an overall impression, however, that patients with Crohn's disease of the small bowel respond better than those with Crohn's colitis or ulcerative colitis. Indeed, a recent controlled trial of total gut rest and parenteral nutrition was unable to show any advantage for this form of treatment and, although the numbers were small, there was no clear-cut difference between the patients with Crohn's colitis and those with ulcerative colitis (Dickinson *et al.*, 1979).

In summary, it may be said that IVN should be used in severely malnourished patients about to undergo major surgery for inflammatory bowel disease. It has a place too in those patients who require urgent or emergency surgery for this condition. It should also be used in some patients with Crohn's disease of the small intestine, particularly where there is evidence of obstruction. In these circumstances, nutritional integrity can be preserved while the gut is rested and time is gained which may allow spontaneous remission. Some workers have had remarkable success with this type of treatment in patients who would otherwise have been subjected to surgery with loss or bypass of a part of the small intestine (Greenberg *et al.*, 1976). It should be remembered, however, that enterocutaneous fistulas arising from an area of bowel in which there is macroscopic evidence of Crohn's disease have little chance of closing spontaneously and surgery is indicated.

Other patients with intestinal inflammation may also receive benefit from gut rest and IVN. There is some evidence that 5-fluorouracil toxicity (stomatitis, nausea and diarrhoea) is less when the gut is rested (Copeland *et al.*, 1975) and patients with radiation enteritis and protein calorie malnutrition may be helped also by a period of such treatment. It is important to remember, however, that an external small bowel fistula arising from an area of irradiated bowel will probably never close and surgical excision or bypass is almost always required.

Applications of IVN when the gastrointestinal tract is unable to cope

Prolonged post-operative ileus, pseudo-obstruction of the colon and familial pseudo-obstruction of the intestine may all require IVN for varying periods while awaiting spontaneous remission. In idiopathic pseudo-obstruction of the intestine (Schuttler *et al.*, 1977) very prolonged periods of IVN may be required and some patients may need to be treated in this way permanently.

Whenever there is an intra-abdominal abscess or septic focus, it is difficult to administer nutrients adequately via the enteral route. Patients with complications of pancreatitis, in particular, come into this category. Prolonged attacks of acute pancreatitis can be associated with rapid deterioration in nutritional state and treatment with total gut rest and IVN appears to be effective.

Pancreatic pseudocysts often resolve spontaneously but those in which this does not occur need surgical drainage. A period of gut rest and IVN 'buys time', allows the cyst wall to mature and thicken, and means that the subsequent surgical procedure is likely to be more straightforward. Pancreatic abscesses, too, need surgical drainage and this may need to be repeated on a number of occasions; without adequate nutritional therapy the associated hypercatabolism and starvation can lead to advanced protein calorie malnutrition.

Contraindications to intravenous nutrition

In many patients requiring nutritional supplementation the gastrointestinal tract is normal and it is much safer to use nasogastric or jejunostomy feeding than to use IVN. Thus it is quite wrong to use IVN in patients with severe malnutrition secondary to a partial oesophageal blockage. In most patients of this type a fine bore nasogastric tube can be passed into the stomach and a formula-defined diet can be continuously infused. Whenever nutritional therapy is required, the clinician must ask if the enteral route can be used. Feeding in this way is just as effective as IVN (Fig. 4.1). The recent introduction of the technique of a fine needle catheter jejunostomy means that this route is also available for use in selected patients in the post-operative period, although this method is also not without its complications (Yeung *et al.*, 1979).

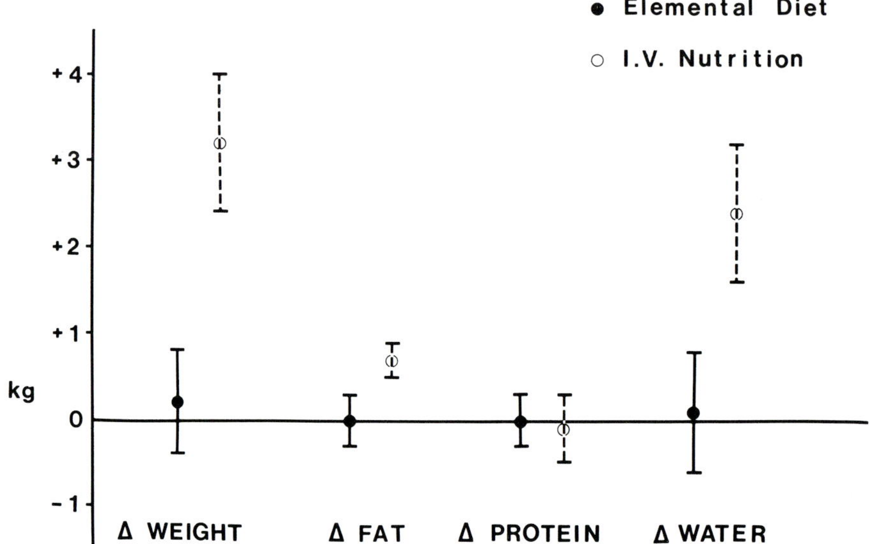

Fig. 4.1. *Changes (mean ± SEM) in body weight, fat, protein and water that occurred in 2 comparable groups of 14 surgical patients over a 2 week period.* The administration of the elemental diet by continuous infusion was comparable to intravenous nutrition in maintaining body protein in these very ill patients.

(from Yeung *et al.*, 1979)

IVN should not be used to prolong life unnecessarily or during periods of cardiovascular instability. It is also contraindicated in the very old and in the very young when there has been total loss of small bowel.

Some clinicians feel that IVN is contraindicated in a patient with continuing sepsis. It is argued that the indwelling catheter will soon become infected, thereby exacerbating the problem. It cannot be too strongly emphasized, however, that patients with continuing sepsis are especially in need of nutritional therapy and that frequent catheter changes (about 2–3 times each week) over a guide wire will minimise the risk of this complication and allow sufficient calories and protein to be given.

ACKNOWLEDGEMENT

Fig. 4.1 is reproduced from *Gastroenterology*, 1979, 77, 652 by permission of the American Gastroenterological Association.

References

Blackett R.L. and Hill G.L. (1978) *Brit. J. Surg.* **65**, 775.

Broviac J.W., Cole J.J. and Scribner B.H. (1973) *Surg. Gynec. Obst.* **136**, 602.

Cannon P.R., Wissler R.W., Woolride R.L. *et al.* (1944) *Ann. Surg.* **120**, 514.

Collins J.P., Oxby C.B. and Hill G.L. (1978) *Lancet*, i, 788.

Copeland E.M., Macfadyen B.V., Lanzotti V.J. *et al.* (1975) *Amer. J. Surg.* **129**, 167.

Dickinson R.J., Ashton M.G., Axon A.T.R. *et al.* (1979) *Gut*, **20**, A445.

Driscoll R.H. and Rosenberg I.H. (1978) *Med. Clin. N. Amer.* **62**, 185.

Dudrick S.J., Wilmore D.W., Vars H.M. *et al.* (1969) *Ann. Surg.* **169**, 974.

Fleming C.R., McGill D.B. and Berkner S. (1977) *Gastroenterology*, **73**, 1077.

Greenberg G.R., Haber G.B. and Jeejeebhoy K.N. (1976) *Gut*, **17**, 828.

Heatley R.V., Hughes L.E., Morgan A. and Okwonga W. (1976) *Lancet*, i, 437.

Hill G.L. (1979) *Med. J. Aust.* **2**, 464.

Hill G.L., Blackett R.L., Pickford I.R. *et al.* (1977) *Brit. J. Surg.* **64**, 894.

Jacobson S. (1972) *Int. Surg.* **57**, 841.

Jeejeebhoy K.N., Langer B., Tsallas G. *et al.* (1976) *Gastroenterology*, **71**, 943.

Ladefoged K. and Jarnum S. (1978) *Brit. med. J.* **2**, 262.

Leading Article (1979) *Lancet*, ii, 507.

Liljedahl S.O. (1972) *Nutr. Metab. (Suppl.)* **14**, 110.

Macfadyen B.V., Dudrick S.J. and Ruberg R.L. (1973) *Surgery*, **74**, 100.

Meakins J.L., Pietsch J.B., Bubenick O. *et al.* (1977) *Ann. Surg.* **186**, 241.

Mullen J.L., Gertner M.H., Buzby G.P. *et al.* (1979) *Arch. Surg.* **114**, 121.

Schuttler M.D., Lowe M.C. and Bill (1977) *Gastroenterology*, **73**, 327.

Solassol C.L., Joyeux H., Etco L. *et al.* (1974) *Ann. Surg.* **179**, 519.

Studley H.O. (1936) *J. Amer. med. Ass.* **106**, 697.

Towne J.B., Hamilton R.F. and Stephenson D.V. (1973) *Amer. J. Surg.* **126**, 714.

Yeung C.K., Smith R.C. and Hill G.L. (1979a), *Gastroenterology*, **77**, 652.

Yeung C.K., Young, G.A., Hackett A.F., Hill G.L. (1979b) *Brit. J. Surg.* **66**, 727.

Young E.A., Heuler N., Russel P. *et al.* (1975) *Gastroenterology*, **69**, 1338.

Chapter 5

Metabolic complications with special reference to folate deficiency

H. F. WOODS

Parenteral feeding is a major therapeutic undertaking, being an attempt to provide all nutrients via the intravenous route. In common with other types of therapy, the potential benefits must be balanced against the risks inherent in the method. Experience has shown that there are a considerable number of complications, which can be divided into two main groups (Woods, 1979);

a) those associated with the need to have a catheter within the circulation, and

b) those mainly reflecting the nature of the nutrients infused.

Among the latter group are the metabolic complications listed in Table 5.1. The list is extensive and the incidence of most complications is unknown. The overall incidence may be difficult to ascertain because the abnormalities may not be detected, either because of inadequate monitoring of the patients or because the underlying disease may mask the symptoms and signs of a particular side-effect.

Analysis of the mechanisms involved in the pathogenesis of metabolic complications reveals that they arise through interactions between the following factors:

(1) The clinical state of the patient;

(2) The nature of the nutrients infused;

(3) The rate of delivery of the infused nutrients.

The present chapter will concentrate on folate deficiency as it exemplifies some of these general mechanisms.

Normal folic acid metabolism

Man normally obtains folic acid in the form of polyglutamates from

Table 5.1. *Metabolic complications of parenteral nutrition*

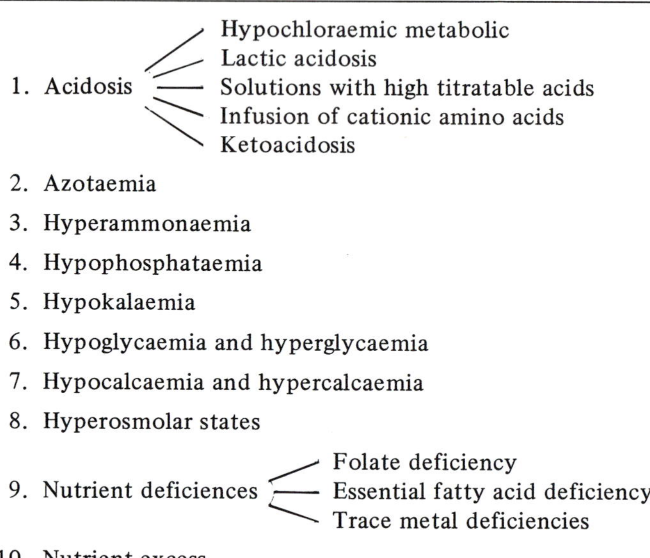

1. Acidosis
   - Hypochloraemic metabolic
   - Lactic acidosis
   - Solutions with high titratable acids
   - Infusion of cationic amino acids
   - Ketoacidosis

2. Azotaemia

3. Hyperammonaemia

4. Hypophosphataemia

5. Hypokalaemia

6. Hypoglycaemia and hyperglycaemia

7. Hypocalcaemia and hypercalcaemia

8. Hyperosmolar states

9. Nutrient deficiences
   - Folate deficiency
   - Essential fatty acid deficiency
   - Trace metal deficiencies

10. Nutrient excess

vegetables, which are a rich source, while milk and meat contain moderate amounts. The vitamin is absorbed in the duodenum and jejunum. Considerable losses occur during the cooking and canning of foods, when between 50 and 100 per cent of the folate content of food may be degraded. The total body stores of folic acid are not accurately known but an average man probably has about three months' reserve of folic acid. The daily requirements are a matter of debate and there is a considerable variation in the recommended daily intake in European countries (Table 5.2).

Folic acid takes part in the reactions involved in nucleic acid synthesis and is important in the maintenance of a normal gut mucosa in addition to its role in haemopoiesis. It also acts as a co-factor in the metabolism of one-carbon (1-C) fragments. The importance of an adequate provision of folic acid during intravenous feeding is clear from a consideration of these functions.

Acute folate deficiency

Wardrop *et al.* (1975) described four surgical patients who developed

Table 5.2. *Recommended folate intake in European countries.* The data refer to adult males and are those listed by the Second European Nutrition Conference (Proceedings, 1976).

Country	Recommended daily intake (μg)
Denmark	400
Federal Germany	400
Italy	200
Spain	200

folate deficiency early in the postoperative period. Three of these had received parenteral nutrition. In all four patients the blood counts and films were normal before the operation. The haematological abnormalities, namely, leukopenia and thrombocytopenia, appeared acutely during a two to seven days period and were accompanied by megaloblastic haemopoiesis in the bone marrow. At the time of diagnosis, the serum folate concentrations were low and in three cases the red cell folate concentration was within normal limits. The serum vitamin B_{12} levels were all normal and the haematological abnormalities were successfully treated by folate administration. In the same year, Ibbotson *et al.* (1975) described two patients who developed folate deficiency during intensive care and who had also received parenteral feeding. Both responded favourably to folate administration.

Green (1977) described two further patients in whom the folate deficiency occurred during parenteral feeding. The biochemical and haematological findings in these cases are shown in Fig. 5.1. Both patients developed pancytopaenia and jaundice, which quickly resolved after folate administration. In one case a bone marrow biopsy revealed megaloblastic haemopoiesis.

A summary of all these cases is shown in Table 5.3 and brief descriptions of two further cases can be found in the literature (Amess *et al.*, 1976; Saary and Hoffbrand, 1976).

The mechanism of production of folate deficiency

The first factor involved in the pathogenesis of the acute folate deficiency is the clinical state of the patients themselves. Many of the indications

Table 5.3. *Acute folate deficiency: a summary of cases.* The data have been abstracted from the articles by Wardrop *et al.* (1975), Ibbotson *et al.* (1975) and Green (1977). In some cases the data recorded in the case-reports are incomplete.

Total number of cases		8
Males		6
Females		2
Age ranges (years): Males		14–70
Females		30 and 74
Diagnoses	Carcinoma of Prostate / Prostatectomy	1
	Crohn's Disease / Colectomy	1
	Carcinoma of stomach / Gastrectomy	1
	Ruptured Oesophagus / Empyema	1
	Crush Injury / Renal Failure	1
	Aortic Aneurysm Repair / Renal Failure	1
	Spina Bifida / Peritonitis	1
	Benign Oesophagal stricture	1
Parenteral Feeding Administered		7
Antimicrobial Therapy		3
Haematological Abnormalities:		
Pancytopenia		6
Anaemia and Thrombocytopenia		1
Megaloblastic marrow		7
Time of appearance of haematological abnormalities:		
Days after admission		
0–10		4
11–20		2
21–30		1
40–50		1
Favourable response to folate administration		4

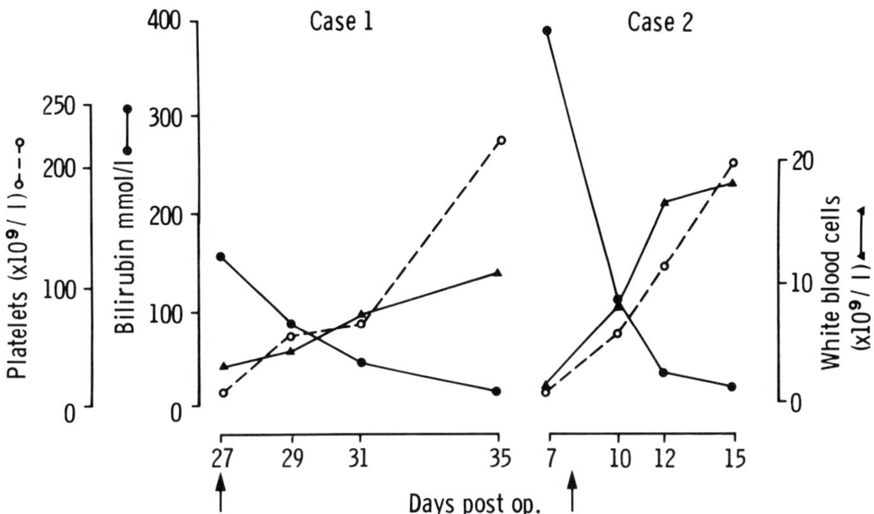

Fig. 5.1. *Folate deficiency in patients fed intravenously — response to therapy.* The figure is plotted using the data of Green (1977) and shows the biochemical and haematological response to an intravenous dose of 9 mg of calcium folinate given at the time indicated by the arrow. Both patients had received intravenous feeding.

for parenteral nutrition stem from disorders of the gastrointestinal tract, especially inflammatory bowel disease. These disorders may result in a poor dietary intake of folate because of a combination of anorexia and poor absorption if those regions of the gut in which folates are absorbed are involved with disease.

Thus Newton *et al.* (1979) found that, prior to the start of parenteral feeding, half of the patients they studied had a low serum folate concentration when compared with an age- and sex-matched control population (Fig. 5.2). All of this low folate group were seriously ill catabolic patients and many had a diagnosis of carcinoma of the stomach or inflammatory bowel disease. In no case, however, was the red cell folate concentration below normal and there were no changes in the blood film suggesting megaloblastic haemopoiesis. All had normal serum vitamin B_{12} concentrations.

The nature of the nutrients infused and their rate of infusion are best considered together. Wardrop *et al.* (1975), after describing their four index cases, went on to study prospectively a group of 25 patients with gastrointestinal disease before and after surgery. These patients were divided in two groups. The first preoperative parenteral feeding with a

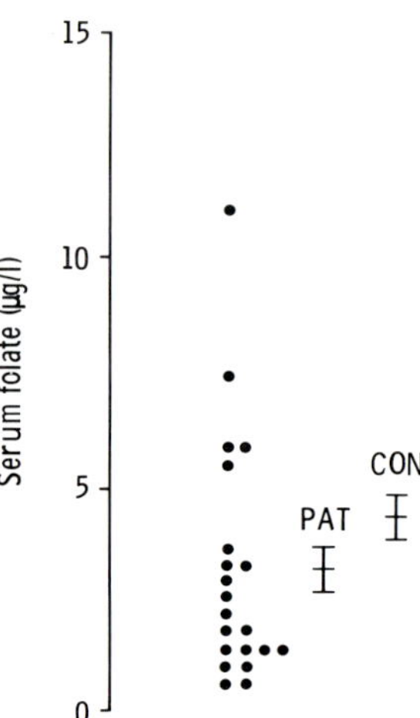

Fig. 5.2. *Serum folate concentrations in patients prior to parenteral feeding.* The data refer to a series of 21 consecutive patients who were about to receive parenteral feeding. Also shown is the mean value ± SEM for this group (PAT) and that for an age- and sex-matched control group (CON). These mean values are significantly different ($p < 0.01$). (After Newton *et al.*, 1979).

sorbitol/amino acid/ethanol mixture in addition to any oral food intake. The second group received no intravenous nutrients. In no patient was there any evidence of folate deficiency before treatment but ten of the thirteen patients who received intravenous nutrition had a marked fall in the serum folate concentrations. In these patients, the folate concentrations returned to normal five days after stopping the intravenous treatment. There were no changes in the serum of the patients who were not fed intravenously and in all subjects the red cell folate concentrations were unaltered. The changes are summarized in Fig. 5.3. Megaloblastic haemopoiesis was found in the marrow of five of the patients whose serum folate remained low for four days or more.

In their discussion, Wardrop *et al.* (1975) listed the factors contributing to folate deficiency in their patients and concluded that the ethanol infused was probably the most important.

Wardrop *et al.* (1977) later attempted to prevent folate deficiency during parenteral nutrition by folate administration. In this study of 30 patients undergoing surgery for gastrointestinal disease, 20 were given 2–3 litres of an amino acid/sorbitol/ethanol mixture for 6–12 days before operation. Of these 20 patients, 10 received the intravenous nutrition alone (Group A), while the other 10 (Group B) were given

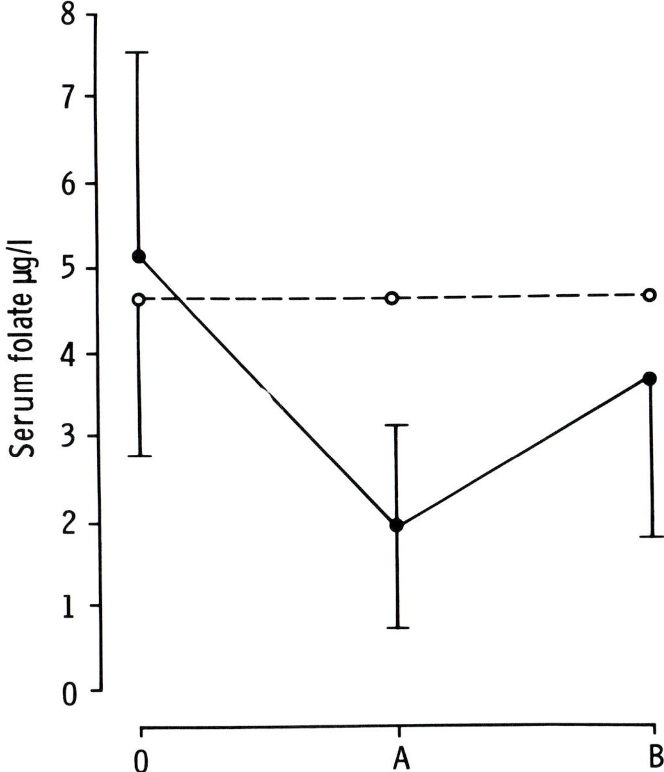

Fig. 5.3. *Serum folate and intravenous nutrition.* The graph shows the serum folate concentrations (mean ± SEM) in two groups of surgical patients. One group (●—●) received parenteral nutrition with an amino acid-sorbitol-ethanol mixture in addition to oral feeding. The second group (O - - - O) received oral feeds alone. The serum folate measurements were performed before treatment (O), after 5 days treatment (A) and five days after treatment had ceased (B). (After Wardrop *et al.*, 1975).

folate supplements in addition. The remaining 10 patients (Group C) received no parenteral feeding or folate therapy and represented a control group.

The red cell folate concentrations did not change significantly in any of the groups but in Groups A and B there was a significant fall in the serum folate concentrations while those in Group C did not change. In Group A the fall in serum folate concentration persisted but in Group B the concentration rapidly returned to normal in the first three post-operative days.

                    H. F. Woods

At operation a bone marrow sample was obtained and the findings are summarized in Table 5.4. Minor marrow abnormalities were present in seven Group A patients and one Group B patient and, of those in Group A with an abnormal marrow, four developed macrocytes in the peripheral blood film during the first postoperative week. Three of the Group A patients with megaloblastic haemopoiesis developed thrombocytopenia, leucopenia or pancytopenia in the postoperative period.

This careful investigation suggested that parenteral feeding was an important cause of acute folate deficiency and, in a later study, the same group showed that cholecystectomy alone was followed by a significant fall of serum folate concentration one day after operation (Smith *et al.*, 1978). They also showed that parenteral nutrition regimens which contained amino acids infused together with sorbitol and ethanol or glucose or fat also resulted in a fall in serum folate concentration (Table 5.5). These investigations suggested that the infusion of ethanol was not the only causative factor.

An alternative mechanism was suggested by Connor *et al.* (1978). They postulated that the acute drop in serum folate concentration in response to the infusion of solutions containing amino acids may be related to the L-methionine content of the solutions. This amino acid is an important source of one-carbon (1-C) units and is a major constituent of all commercially available amino acid mixtures. Because folate derivatives are involved as co-factors in normal 1-C unit metabolism an excess of L-methionine could influence folate homeostasis by increasing the metabolic 'demand' for folate.

In this study five healthy volunteers were given an oral supplement of 8 grams of L-methionine per day in divided doses continued for five days. The dose was chosen to be similar to that given via the

Table 5.4. *Bone marrow and blood film findings after parenteral feeding (Based on the data of Wardrop* et al., *1977).*

Patient Group	Type of feeding	No. with abnormal marrow	No. with abnormal blood film
A	Parenteral	7/10	4/10*
B	Parenteral + folate	1/10	0/10
C	Oral	0/8	0/10

*These four patients all had an abnormal marrow at operation

Table 5.5. *The influence of the type of regimen on serum folate concentrations during parenteral feeding.* The data have been extracted from the data of Wardrop *et al.* (1975, 1977) and Smith *et al.* (1978). The fall in serum folate should be compared with that which occurs 24 hours after cholecystectomy (37%, according to Smith *et al.* 1978). Also included is the L-methionine content of the solutions used (ABPI Data Sheet Compendium, 1979).

Pre-operative Treatment regimen	% fall in serum folate concentration after 48 h therapy	L-methionine content of the amino acid mixture used (g/l)
Aminoplex 5 alone	80	2·4
Aminoplex 5 + Intralipid	63	2·4
Aminoplex 5 + folate supplements	65	2·4
Aminoplex 14 + glucose	66	6·4
Vamin N + glucose	54	1·9
Glucose–saline	0	0

intravenous route by Wardrop *et al.* (1975). The serum folate concentrations fell significantly one day after starting L-methionine supplements (Fig. 5.4) and remained low throughout the treatment. No change was seen in the red cell folate concentration. The plasma L-methionine concentrations rose to a level similar to that reported by Smits and Wells (1975) as occurring in patients who were receiving 7·2 g of L-methionine daily as part of an intravenous feeding regimen consisting of the same solution used by Wardrop *et al.* (1975).

Changes in the blood film were slight, comprising a small rise in red cell volume and a drop in total red cell count on day four, and a rise in the white cell count on day five. Two subjects later repeated the study with oral folate supplements (5 mg/day) which prevented the fall in serum folate concentration.

This work showed that the serum folate concentration fell acutely when subjects eating a normal diet were given a L-methionine supplement and thus the experimental conditions differed from those during intravenous feeding. However, the L-methionine supplement probably disturbed the normal relationship between folate and L-methionine in a manner similar to that which occurs in patients given intravenous L-methionine without folate or in subjects with depleted folate stores. The mechanism is unclear. The L-methionine loading probably increased

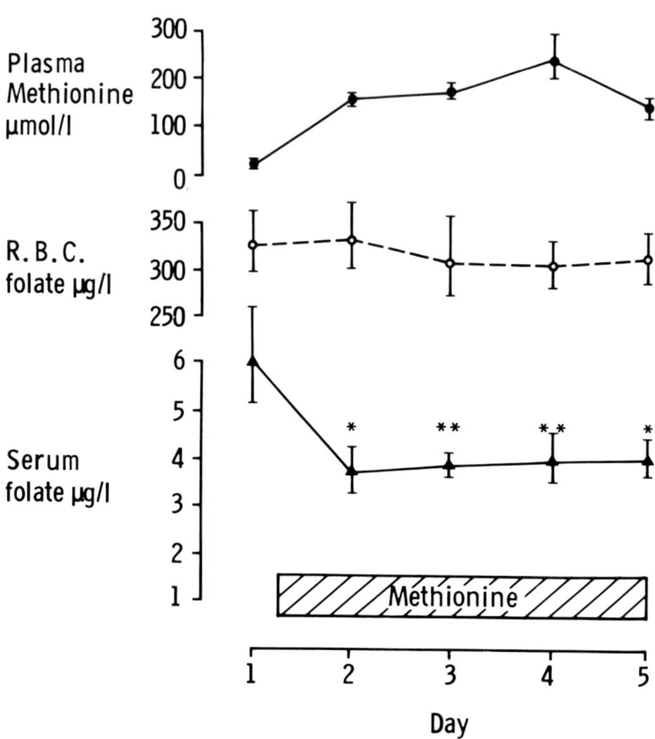

Fig. 5.4. *The effect of L-methionine loading on serum folate concentrations in normal man.* Concentrations of serum folate, red cell folate and L-methionine (mean ± SEM) in five subjects during oral loading with L-methionine (8 g daily). Serum folate concentrations significantly different from day 1: $*p < 0.05$, $**p < 0.005$. (After Connor *et al.*, 1978).

the amount of reduced folates such as methyltetrahydrofolate in serum as suggested by Krebs and Hems (1976). These chemical forms of folate are only weakly bound to serum folate-binding protein and thus are more available for redistribution via cellular uptake (Waxman, 1975).

Taken together the work reviewed above would suggest that the two main factors involved in the production of acute folate deficiency are the depletion of folate in the tissues and body fluids of patients being fed intravenously before treatment was started and a disturbance in folate metabolism caused by the infusion of amino acid mixtures. The rate of infusion of L-methionine may be a critical factor although L-methionine is only one of several compounds (such as histidine and serine) used in parenteral nutrition which take part in 1-C fragment metabolism. The normal L-methionine requirement in man is about

2 g per day and infusion of 7 or 8 g per day far exceeds the capacity of normal subjects to metabolize the amino acid via normal pathways (Burger, 1979), thus favouring the alternative routes of metabolism and disposition.

Treatment with antimicrobials, cytotoxic agents and anti-epileptic drugs may also modify the metabolism of folate and these classes of drug are frequently used in the patients who need nutritional support. In addition, it would be wrong to dismiss ethanol infusion as being unimportant. Although the mechanisms of the toxic effects of this compound on the bone marrow are not clear, it can cause a large fall in serum folate concentrations (Eichner and Hillman, 1973).

Conclusions and therapeutic recommendations

It is not possible to state the overall incidence of folate deficiency induced by parenteral feeding but Wardrop *et al.* (1977) state that in their experience the frequency of haematological toxicity of infused amino acid/sorbitol/ethanol mixtures given without folate supplements is more than 10%.

The facts discussed here have implications for patient management. Firstly, they underline the need for comprehensive metabolic screening before parenteral feeding is started and its continuation during the therapy (Newton *et al.*, 1979, 1980). Secondly, if the rate of L-methionine infusion is a major factor, treatment with 5 mg of folic acid per day was more than adequate in preventing the fall in serum folate concentration caused by L-methionine loading in normal subjects. Wretlind (1974) has recommended a daily folate supplement for patients receiving parenteral nutrition of about 200 μg for a 70 kg adult. This may be inadequate when it is remembered that many of those being fed have depleted stores of folate before parenteral feeding is started. On this basis Connor *et al.* (1978) have suggested that an initial dose of 10 mg is given to replenish body stores followed by 0·5 mg daily. Caution must be exercised because, as Wardrop *et al.* (1977) have pointed out, the dose of folic acid should not be large enough to mask the haematological signs of incipient vitamin B_{12} deficiency or to precipitate neurological damage.

Finally, the inclusion of large amounts of L-methionine in the formulation of commercial amino acid mixtures can be questioned, particularly when it is borne in mind that the daily requirement for this amino acid is greatly exceeded in many regimens that provide a dose of nitrogen sufficient to meet the needs of the catabolic malnourished patient.

ACKNOWLEDGEMENTS

The data in Tables 4 and 5 and Figures 1, 3 and 4 are reproduced by permission of the Editors of The Lancet, the British Medical Journal, the Postgraduate Medical Journal and the British Journal of Haematology.

References

Amess J.A.L., Burman J.F. and Mollin D.L. (1976) *Brit. med. J.* i, 525.

Bürger U. (1977) *Infusionstherapie,* **4**, 273.

Connor H., Newton D.J., Preston F.E. and Woods H.F. (1978) *Postgrad. med. J.* **54**, 318.

Eichner E.R. and Hillman R.S. (1973) *J. clin. Invest.* **52**, 584.

Green P.J. (1977) *Lancet,* i, 814.

Ibbotson R.M., Colvin B.T. and Colvin M.P. (1975) *Brit. med. J.* **iv**, 145.

Krebs H.A. and Hems R. (1976) *Advances in Enzyme Regulation,* **14**, 493.

Newton D.J., Clark R.G., Woods H.F. and Connor H. (1979) *Proc. Nutr. Soc.* **38**(2), A-74.

Newton D.J., Clark R.G. and Woods H.F. (1980) *Proc. Nutr. Soc.* **39**, 141.

Proceedings of the Second European Nutrition Conference (Munich 1976) Zöllner N., Wolfram G. and Keller Ch. (1977) *Nutr. Metab.* **21**, 251.

Saary M. and Hoffbrand A.V. (1976) *Brit. med. J.* i, 461.

Smith R.C., Tennant G.B., Williams C.A. and Wardrop C.A.J. (1978) *Brit. J. Surg.* **65**, 364.

Smits B.J. and Wells F.E. (1975) *Clin. Trials,* **12**, (Suppl. I), 186.

Wardrop C.A.J., Heatley R.V., Tennant G.B. and Hughes L.E. (1975) *Lancet,* ii, 640.

Wardrop C.A.J., Lewis M.H., Tennant G.B., Williams R.H.P. and Hughes L.E. (1977) *Brit. J. Haematol.* **37**, 521.

Waxman S. (1975) *Brit. J. Haematol.* **29**, 23.

Wretlind A. (1974). In *Parenteral Nutrition in Acute Metabolic Illness.* ed. Lee H.A. Academic Press, London and New York.

Woods H.F. (1979). In *Topics in Therapeutics 5.* ed. Davis D.M. and Rawlins M.D. Pitman Medical, Tunbridge Wells.

Chapter 6
Its use in inflammatory conditions

GAVIN ROYLE

Inflammation is defined as the response of living tissues to injury. The response is both local and general. The local response is classically described as rubor, calor, dolor, tumor and loss of function. The general response includes changes in the blood, cardiovascular system, organs and metabolism. Inflammation may be acute or chronic. Examples of the former are septicaemia and thermal burns. Examples of chronic inflammation are intra-abdominal abscesses which have been present for a week or more, and inflammatory bowel disease. Patients suffering from inflammation, whether acute or chronic, may require parenteral nutrition. However, inflammation is a natural defence mechanism and it would appear wise to try to understand the metabolic changes that occur as a result of inflammation before the metabolism is further altered by the infusion of various substrates, electrolytes, trace elements and vitamins.

Metabolic changes in acute inflammation

Cuthbertson (1932) made the original observation that accidental injury is followed by increased nitrogen loss in the urine, a loss which may be greater than 20 g of nitrogen a day. It is generally agreed that the nitrogen excreted in the urine comes from muscle. Recent work has shown that the negative nitrogen balance following injury results from decreased protein synthesis as well as from increased protein breakdown (O'Keefe *et al.*, 1974; Waterlow *et al.*, 1977). Mobilization of muscle protein after injury is useful in providing 'building blocks' for tissue repair as well as carbon skeletons for glucose synthesis. If this catabolic response continues, however, it is not of benefit to the patient.

Factors that initiate or maintain the catabolic response are the central nervous system (Stoner, 1976) and the endocrine system (Wilmore, 1976). The nature and severity of the injury, the environmental temperature, and the nutritional status of the patient are factors which modify the metabolic response to injury (Cuthbertson, 1976). Recently it has also been observed that nitrogen and 3-methyl histidine excretion are inversely related to blood ketone—body concentrations after injury (Smith *et al.*, 1975; Williamson *et al.*, 1977). Urinary excretion of 3-methyl histidine is a useful indicator of muscle protein breakdown as 3-methyl histidine is a product of actin and myosin breakdown and is not resynthesized.

Glucose turnover is increased after burns (Wolfe *et al.*, 1977) and the well-known hyperglycaemia after injury may result from increased hepatic release of glucose rather than decreased peripheral uptake of glucose.

Metabolic changes in chronic inflammation

In contrast to the increased catabolism of acute inflammation (Table 6.1), the metabolic response to chronic inflammation is subdued. Urinary nitrogen and 3-methyl histidine excretion are not increased, the urinary nitrogen excretion in chronic inflammation usually bring less than 10 g/day (Royle, 1979). Glucose turnover is probably reduced rather than increased. In contrast to the hyperglycaemic response after acute injury (Elia *et al.*, 1979), basal blood glucose concentration is not increased and intravenous infusion of the hepatic glucose precursor, galactose, results in only small increases in blood glucose and

Table 6.1. *Metabolic changes in acute and chronic inflammation*

Metabolic changes	Acute inflammation	Chronic inflammation
Glucose turnover	Increased	Reduced
Muscle protein synthesis	Reduced	Reduced
Muscle protein breakdown	Unchanged or increased	Unchanged or reduced
Lipolysis	Increased	Increased
Ketogenesis	Increased, unchanged or reduced	Increased

lactate concentrations in patients with chronic inflammation (Royle *et al.*, 1978a and b) (Table 6.2). Chronic sepsis is also associated with hyperketonaemia and low blood alanine concentrations. Alanine is the major glucogenic amino acid in man and the low blood alanine concentration in chronic sepsis, unlike the increased blood concentration of alanine following acute injury (Smith *et al.*, 1975), probably results from decreased muscle release rather than increased hepatic uptake (Royle *et al.*, 1978c). The experimental infusion of ketone bodies in man has been shown to reduce urinary nitrogen excretion and to decrease blood alanine concentrations (Sherwin *et al.*, 1975).

The metabolic response of chronic inflammation is thus different from that of acute inflammation. The actual cause is uncertain but malnutrition is likely to be an important factor. There is strong anthropometric and biochemical evidence that patients with chronic abscesses or inflammatory bowel disease are malnourished (Tables 6.3 and 6.4). Experimental malnutrition is known to reduce the catabolic response to injury (Fleck and Munro, 1963).

There are several causes for malnutrition in patients with chronic inflammation. Patients who have intra-abdominal abscesses have often undergone major surgery, may be losing protein from sinuses or fistulae, are anorexic, and may not receive enough calories and protein, either orally or parenterally. Similarly, patients with inflammatory bowel disease may have a poor oral food intake due to anorexia, operation, or the therapeutic withdrawal of oral food to 'rest' the intestine. Patients

Table 6.2. *Glucogenesis in chronic inflammation. Response to intravenous galactose (20g).* Values shown as the mean ± SEM. (Adapted from Royle *et al.* 1978b).

	Galactose T½ (min)	Basal blood glucose (mmol/l)	Glucose increase (mmol/l)	Basal blood Lactate (mmol/l)	Lactate increase (mmol/l)
Control (n = 9)	13·9 ± 1·0	5·01 ± 0·19	0·69 ± 0·11	0·65 ± 0·09	0·22 ± 0·08
Chronic sepsis (n = 7)	17·1 ± 1·9	5·17 ± 0·19	0·36 ± 0·09*	0·69 ± 0·12	0·05 ± 0·02
Recovered septic (n = 4)	13·6 ± 3·0	5·30 ± 0·23	0·85 ± 0·14	0·59 ± 0·03	0·16 ± 0·09

*p < 0·05 compared with control.

Table 6.3. *Evidence for malnutrition in chronic inflammation as shown by the effects of chronic intra-abdominal abscess.* Values shown as the mean ± SEM. (Adapted from Royle *et al.*, 1978b).

	Age (yr)	Weight (kg)	Weight Loss (%)	Plasma Albumin (g/l)	Plasma Cholesterol (mmol/l)	Hb (g%)
Control (n = 9)	60 ± 2	69 ± 5	3 ± 5	40 ± 1	5·3 ± 0·5	13·6 ± 1·3
Septic (n = 7)	63 ± 3	60 ± 4	21 ± 5*	29 ± 3**	2·6 ± 5**	11·7 ± 1·4**
Recovered septic (n = 4)	56 ± 4	56 ± 4	21 ± 7*	38 ± 1	5·0 ± 0·08	13·4 ± 0·7

*$P<0.05$, **$P<0.01$ compared with control.

with inflammatory bowel disease may have malabsorption due to the diseased bowel, intestinal resection or the presence of fistulae. These patients may also suffer from a protein-losing enteropathy or be subject to the increased metabolic demands of operation or acute infection. It is well known that malnutrition predisposes to infection and that infection makes the results of malnutrition worse (Scrimshaw, 1966). A vicious circle may thus be induced. The resulting protein-calorie malnutrition may be of the marasmus or kwashiorkor type or a combination of both (Leading Article, *Lancet,* 1970). Marasmus is characterized by loss of weight whereas, in kwashiorkor, there is oedema and low plasma albumin concentration.

Parenteral nutrition and inflammation

As acute and chronic inflammation induce different metabolic responses, patients with inflammatory disease who require parenteral feeding should have a regimen suited to their particular needs. The degree of catabolism is the key factor. There are also other factors which should be considered before prescribing a regimen. Patients with inflammatory disease are often severely ill, may be considerably malnourished, and often have poor peripheral veins. This means that they are usually best treated by total parenteral nutrition via a central venous catheter rather than by 'protein-sparing' isotonic amino acid

Table 6.4. *Evidence for malnutrition in chronic inflammation as shown by the effects of inflammatory bowel disease.* Values shown as the mean ± SD. AMC = Arm muscle circumference. (Adapted from Hill *et al.*, 1977).

	Weight loss (%)	AMC (cm)	Plasma albumin (g/l)	Plasma transferrin (mg %)	Plasma pre-albumin (mg %)	Hb (g %)
Control (n = 15)	0	26·0 ± 2·4	43·1 ± 2·2	283 ± 25	29·5 ± 4·2	14·7 ± 1·4
Elective surgery (n = 12)	6·5 ± 7·2	25·3 ± 3·9	41·7 ± 5·4	242 ± 94	26·0 ± 9·5	12·1 ± 2·0**
Acute attack (n = 12)	9·8 ± 5·8	26·1 ± 4·6	41·7 ± 6·8	229 ± 110	24·7 ± 11·9	10·9 ± 2·2***
Urgent surgery (n = 10)	12·4 ± 9·6	25·0 ± 3·4	38·5 ± 5·3*	177 ± 67***	19·1 ± 13·0	11·5 ± 1·6***
Post-surgery complications (n = 9)	24·4 ± 8·0	20·1 ± 1·7***	35·4 ± 5·6**	139 ± 71***	10·9 ± 7·0***	11·7 ± 0·7***

*$P<0.05$, **$P<0.01$, ***$P<0.001$ compared with control.

solutions administered via peripheral veins (Blackburn *et al.*, 1973). Total parenteral nutrition is the intravenous infusion of the correct amounts of all the substances that would normally be absorbed by the gastrointestinal tract.

Parenteral nutrition in acute inflammation

It is probably not wise or practicable for the initial treatment of a patient suffering from septic shock to include parenteral feeding. The first step must be to restore normal cardiovascular function. This usually means the infusion of plasma and expanders rather than substrate solutions. However, as soon as a stable cardiovascular status is achieved parenteral nutrition may be commenced. The main aim is to reduce the catabolic response and to prevent or correct any metabolic deficiencies (Table 6.5). The use of insulin is likely to be beneficial, as insulin opposes the action of the catabolic hormones, such as catecholamines, glucagon and cortisol, the secretion of which is increased in acute inflammation. Insulin also has anabolic effects, as it promotes protein synthesis and decreases hepatic glucose release (Craig *et al.*, 1961). It may also improve cardiac output (Clowes *et al.*, 1974). In clinical practice, intravenous insulin and glucose have been shown to reduce urinary nitrogen excretion in hypercatabolic patients who excrete more than 15 g of urinary nitrogen per day (Hinton *et al.*, 1971; Woolfson *et al.*, 1979). Sufficient electrolytes, particularly potassium, must also be given intravenously. A suggested regimen is shown in Table 6.6. Soluble insulin should be infused intravenously by a syringe pump to keep the blood glucose concentration in the range 7–10 mmol/l. In acute injury, fat does not appear to be such an efficient energy source as glucose and is therefore best avoided (Long *et al.*, 1977; McDougal *et al.*, 1977). Hyperlactataemia is present

Table 6.5. *Aims of parenteral feeding in acute inflammation*

(1) Reduce catabolism

(2) Maintain electrolyte & fluid balance

(3) Prevent metabolic deficiencies

(4) Improve tissue perfusion

(5) Safety

Table 6.6. *Suggested regimen for parenteral feeding in acute inflammation*

Glucose	500 g	
Insulin	As necessary	per 24 h
Amino acids	14 g N	

+ Electrolytes, minerals, trace elements, vitamins, fatty acids.

in the critically ill patient and a lactate load is only slowly removed (Royle and Kettlewell, 1978). Sorbitol, fructose and ethanol, which may cause lactic acidosis, should therefore be avoided (Woods and Alberti, 1972).

Glucose is the ideal calorie source in the patient with acute inflammation. However, it should be noted that the intravenous infusion of large amounts of glucose (>60 kcal/kg/24 h) may lead to the increased deposition of fat in the liver in ill patients (Messing *et al.*, 1977; Burke *et al.*, 1979). Sufficient nitrogen should be provided as L-amino acids to keep the patient in positive nitrogen balance. While it is generally agreed that there should be a 'good' balance of essential and non-essential amino acids, the best combination is not yet known.

Parenteral nutrition in chronic inflammation

These patients are usually in a stable cardiovascular state but are malnourished. The correction of malnutrition, which may be severe, is the main aim (Table 6.7). In those patients with chronic inflammation who cannot take food by the intestinal route, it would seem sensible to provide a well-balanced diet by the intravenous route. A suggested regimen is shown in Table 6.8, which is similar to the normal U.K. oral diet (Hollingsworth, 1979) and supplies both glucose and fat in appro-

Table 6.7. *Metabolic aims of parenteral feeding in chronic inflammation*

1. Prevent or correct metabolic deficiencies
2. Correct nitrogen balance
3. Maintain fluid and electrolyte balance
4. Safety

Table 6.8. *Parenteral feeding in chronic inflammation*

	Suggested regimen	
Glucose	250 g	
Fat	100 g	per 24 h
Amino acids	14 g N	

\+ Electrolytes, trace elements, minerals and vitamins. Albumin and blood as indicated.

priate amounts. It is now well known that trace element deficiencies may occur in patients who require parenteral nutrition. These include zinc, copper, chromium and even selenium (Leading Article, *Brit. med. J.* 1978; van Rij *et al.*, 1979). Deficiencies of folic acid, vitamin C and essential fatty acids should also be prevented. Intramuscular vitamin K and B_{12} may also be indicated. Deficiencies of fat-soluble vitamins do not appear to be so common and, if given in excess, fat-soluble vitamins may be dangerous; however, as a general rule, it is better to prevent metabolic deficiencies than to treat established deficiency syndromes. The intravenous infusion of albumin may be necessary in the short term as the rate of synthesis of albumin is comparatively slow. The use of fat (intralipid) as a calorie source in malnourished patients has several advantages. These include the provision of essential fatty acids, a source of phosphate, and a medium via which fat-soluble vitamins may be given intravenously. Due to its high energy value (9 kcal/g), fat also enables a reduction in the overall volume of fluid and the amount of glucose which needs to be given. The regimen in Table 6.8 contains 250 g glucose and does not require exogenous insulin when given from a 3-litre bag over 24 hours. This means easier nursing and monitoring, with little chance of rebound hypoglycaemia, hyperglycaemia or a hyperosmolar state, which may occur if large amounts of glucose are infused. There is also some evidence that excess insulin may not be beneficial in malnourished patients, due to its antilipolytic effect (Blackburn *et al.*, 1973). Contra-indications to the use of fat are few but include liver failure, coagulopathies and hyperlipidaemia (Wretlind, 1977). Intralipid is, however, expensive.

Patients with inflammatory bowel disease are often candidates for parenteral nutrition. Parenteral nutrition may be used as a primary treatment for an acute attack of inflammatory bowel disease, for the treatment of fistulae and for the treatment of the short bowel syndrome. Parenteral nutrition may also be used as an adjunct to surgery. Patients with severe inflammatory bowel disease often require parenteral nutrition, surgery and steroid therapy in combination (Mullen *et al.*, 1978; Driscoll & Rosenberg, 1978). The regimen in Table 6.8 is particularly suitable for patients receiving steroid therapy, as half the calories are supplied as fat and, even with high doses of steroids, exogenous insulin is rarely required to control blood glucose concentrations. The results of this regimen have been studied in Oxford in 17 patients with inflammatory bowel disease who were either suffering from an acute attack or undergoing urgent surgery. All received intravenous prednisolone 21-phosphate (10–64 mg/day) starting 24 hours before and

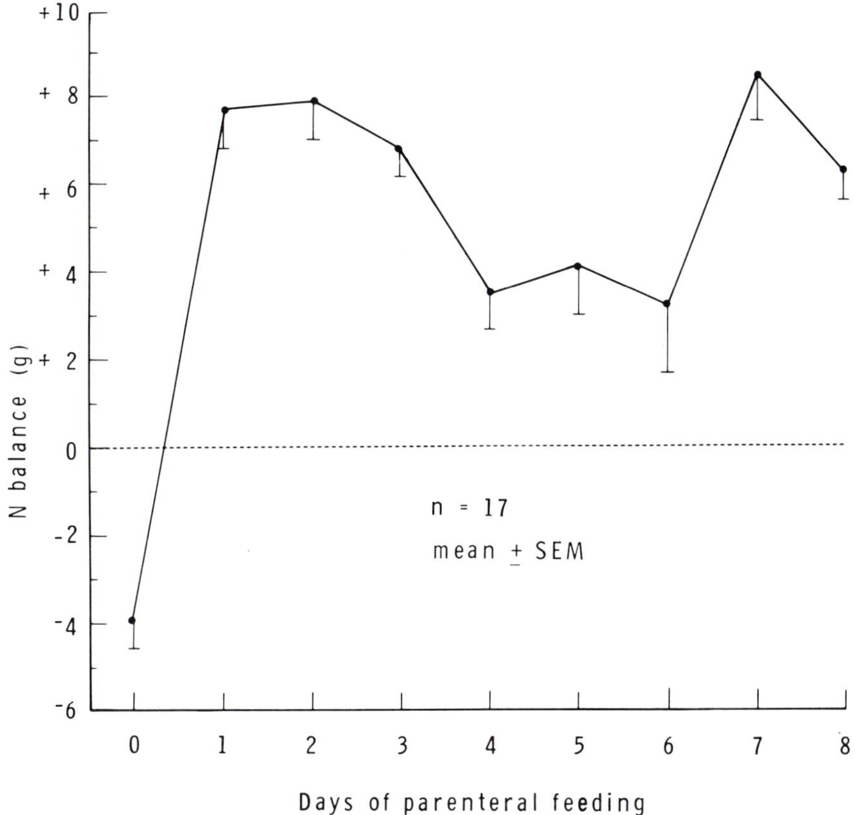

Fig. 6.1. *Nitrogen balance in patients with inflammatory bowel disease (Table 6.9) who received parenteral nutrition with a standard regimen (Table 6.8) for chronic inflammatory conditions.*

 Gavin Royle

continuing throughout the period of parenteral feeding. A positive nitrogen balance was easily achieved in all patients, nitrogen excretion being less than 5 g/day prior to the start of parenteral feeding (Fig. 6.1). There were no metabolic complications. Blood glucose concentration did increase (Fig. 6.2), but only one patient required insulin to prevent glycosuria. Fat was infused over 8–12 hours and persistent hyperlipidaemia was not found. These results are similar to those of Jeejeebhoy *et al.* (1976) who reported that using fat as an energy source in the parenteral nutrition of patients with various gastrointestinal disorders resulted in a positive nitrogen balance.

Results of parenteral nutrition in inflammatory bowel disease

Sixty per cent of patients with an acute attack of ulcerative colitis will achieve remission of symptoms with a five-day course of intravenous steroids and parenteral nutrition (Truelove *et al.*, 1978). Similarly, loss of body weight can be prevented in patients with ulcerative colitis and in those with Crohn's disease who suffer from an acute attack or require urgent surgery (Mullen *et al.*, 1978; Royle *et al.*, 1980). Postoperative surgical complications may also be reduced (Collins *et al.*, 1978). An increase in body weight is hard to achieve. Parenteral feeding has revolutionized the treatment of many gastrointestinal fistulae (MacFadyen *et al.*, 1973). However, Crohn's disease fistulae may be refrac-

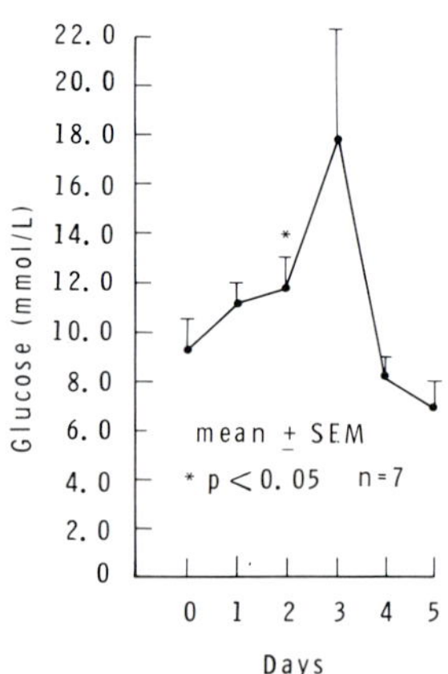

Fig. 6.2. *Blood glucose concentrations in patients with inflammatory bowel disease who received parenteral nutrition. *p<0·05 compared with Day 0 (Prefeeding).*

tory to parenteral nutrition alone: 89—100 % of Crohn's fistulae have been reported to be healed by a combination of surgery and parenteral feeding, whereas only 28—40% were healed by parenteral nutrition alone (Eisenberg *et al.*, 1974; Mullen *et al.*, 1978; Driscoll and Rosenberg, 1978). This emphasizes that the surgical rules of fistula management certainly apply to inflammatory bowel disease: distal obstruction should be relieved, an epithelialized track excised, a foreign body or carcinoma removed, and an adjacent abscess drained. Parenteral nutrition may be administered for as long as a patient cannot absorb a proper diet by the intestinal route, provided there are no complications. A few patients with inflammatory bowel disease are ultimately candidates for home parenteral feeding (Chapter 7).

Conclusions

Major advances have been made in the technique of administration of parenteral nutrition in the last few years. Improvements include a choice of non-toxic substrates and amino acid solutions and technical developments in the way these solutions are given such as 3-litre bags and buried silastic catheters. Advantage should be taken of them in the parenteral feeding of patients with inflammatory disease.

The inflammatory response may be acute or chronic, the catabolic response of acute inflammation undergoing adaptation to become the subdued response of chronic inflammation. This results in a normal or low (< 15 gN/24 h) urinary nitrogen excretion in patients with persistent intra-abdominal abscesses or inflammatory bowel disease, which is different from the large increases in nitrogen excretion found in patients with acute injury. A high-glucose/insulin/amino acid regimen will reduce the negative nitrogen balance in patients with acute inflammation. The correction of malnutrition in patients with chronic inflammation is the main objective when parenteral feeding is indicated. A regimen which provides half the non-nitrogen calories as fat and half as glucose will result in a positive nitrogen balance in these patients. Such a regimen is safe, free of metabolic complications and easy to administer.

Parenteral nutrition is a major therapeutic advance but it is expensive and still subject to technical complications. Further studies are needed to define its indications and benefits in acute and chronic inflammatory conditions.

References

Blackburn G.L. *et al.* (1973) *Amer. J. Surg.* **125**, 447.

Burke J.F. *et al.* (1979) *Ann. Surg.* **190**, 274.

Clowes G.H.A. *et al.* (1974) *Ann. Surg.* **179**, 684.

Collins J.P. *et al.* (1978) *Lancet,* **i**, 788.

Craig J.W. *et al.* (1961) *Metabolism,* **10**, 212.

Cuthbertson D.P. (1932) *Quart. J. Med.* **1**, 233.

Cuthbertson D. (1976). In *Metabolism and the Response to Injury,* eds. Wilkinson A.W. and Cuthbertson D. p. 29. Pitman, London.

Driscoll R.H. and Rosenberg I.H. (1978) *Med. Clin. Amer.* **62**, 185.

Elia M. *et al.* (1979) *Clin. Sci.* **57**, 249.

Eisenberg H.W. *et al.* (1974) *Dis. Colon Rectum.* **17**, 469.

Fleck A. and Munro H.N. (1963) *Metabolism,* **12**, 783.

Hill G.L. *et al.* (1977) *Brit. J. Surg.* **64**, 894.

Hinton P. *et al.* (1971) *Lancet,* **i**, 767.

Hollingsworth D.F. (1979) *J. hum. Nutr.* **33**, 211.

Jeejeebhoy K.N. *et al.* (1976) *J. clin. Invest.* **57**, 125.

Leading Article (1970) *Lancet,* **ii**, 302.

Leading Article (1978) *Brit. med. J.* **ii**, 914.

Long, J.M. *et al.* (1977) *Ann. Surg.* **185**, 417.

MacFadyen B. V. Jr. *et al.* (1973) *Surgery,* **74**, 100.

McDougal W.S. *et al.* (1977) *Surg. Gynec. Obst.* **145**, 408.

Messing B. *et al.* (1977) *Gastroenterol. Clin. Biol.* **1**, 1015.

Mullen J.L. *et al.* (1978) *Ann. Surg.* **187**, 523.

O'Keefe S.J.D. *et al.* (1974) *Lancet,* **ii**, 1035.

Royle G.T. and Kettlewell M.G.W. (1978) *Brit. J. Surg.* **65**, 661.

Royle G. *et al.* (1978a) *Clin. Sci. Mol. Med.* **54**, 107.

Royle G. *et al.* (1978b) *Clin. Sci. Mol. Med.* **55**, 199.

Royle G. *et al.* (1978c) *Brit. J. Surg.* **65**, 363.

Royle G.T. (1979) *Metabolism in Sepsis and Malnutrition.* M.S. Thesis, London University.

Royle G.T. *et al.* (1980) (unpublished).

Scrimshaw N.S. (1966) *Fed. Proc.* **25**, 1679.

Sherwin R.S. *et al.* (1975) *J. clin. Invest.* **55**, 1382.

Smith R. *et al.* (1975) *Lancet,* **i**, 1.

Stoner H.B. (1976). In *Metabolism and the Response to Injury,* eds. Wilkinson A.W. and Cuthbertson D. p. 179, Pitman, London.

Truelove S.C. *et al.* (1978) *Lancet,* **ii**, 1086.

van Rij A.M. *et al.* (1979) *Amer. J. clin. Nutr.* **32**, 2076.

Waterlow J.C. *et al.* (1977) *Amer. J. clin. Nutr.* **30**, 1333.

Williamson D.H. *et al.* (1977) *Clin Sci. Mol. Med.* **52**, 527.

Wilmore D.W. (1976) *Surg. Clin. N. Amer.* **56**, 999.

Wolfe R.R. *et al.* (1977) *Surg. Gynec. Obst.* **144**, 359.

Woods H.F. and Alberti K.G.M.M. (1972) *Lancet,* **ii**, 1354.

Woolfson A.M.J. *et al.* (1979) *N. Engl. J. Med.* **300**, 14.

Wretlind A. (1977). In *Current concepts in parenteral nutrition,* ed. Greep, Soetors, Wesdorp, Phaf and Fischer. Martinus Nijhoff, The Hague.

Chapter 7
Home parenteral feeding

H. JOYEUX and Cl. SOLASSOL

Ambulatory parenteral nutrition is a particular mode of parenteral nutrition which we are able to perform as a result of technical progress and a new conception of nutritive solutions (Joyeux and Astruc, 1980). The objectives of ambulatory parenteral nutrition during the course of intravenous feeding are to encourage the development of muscle, to avoid an excess synthesis of fat and to maintain a good nutritional status. Thus it is possible to obtain optimum nutritional status with the rehabilitation of the musculo-skeletal system. All patients undergoing total or partial parenteral nutrition in our unit are equipped with the 'special' system which allows ambulatory nutrition whenever the physician permits it and whenever the patient can handle it and desires it. Only a few patients (58 out of a total of 3125 patients dealt with during the period 1972—1979) were chosen and prepared for home nutrition according to medical indications and specific criteria of selection. In this chapter we shall consider only patients who underwent home parenteral nutrition for more than one month (35 days to 1,927 days).

Theoretical justification of ambulatory nutrition

During prolonged body rest, there is a decrease in muscle phospholipids and glycogen. The lipids are converted into fatty acids and accumulate in the fatty tissues in the form of triglycerides. The glucose is transformed into glycogen in the liver and into lipids which are transported into the fatty tissues. The catabolism of muscle proteins increases the urinary excretion of nitrogen. Muscular inactivity leads to osteoporosis with an increase in the urinary excretion of calcium. Physical activity facilitates the fixation of calcium by the bone and prevents osteoporosis.

During physical activity there is an increase in the quantity of phospholipids in the muscle. The triglycerides of the fatty tissue are converted into fatty acids and then into phospholipids by the liver. Physical exercise, if it is sufficiently intense and prolonged, is accompanied by important changes in the lipid balance, such as a moderate decrease in total cholesterol, a definite decrease in triglycerides, low density lipoproteins and LDL cholesterol, and a marked increase in HDL cholesterol. The glucose is used for the formation of muscle glycogen and the production of energy in the form of ATP. The branched-chain aminoacids are used in the synthesis of myoglobin and muscle proteins and the number of myofibrils is increased. (For the scientific basis of this section, see Byrne *et al.*, 1979; Enger *et al.*, 1977; Felig and Wahren, 1971; Heizer and Orringer, 1977; Jeejeebhoy *et al.*, 1976; Joyeux and Astruc, 1980; Miller and Ivey, 1979; Powell-Tuck *et al.*, 1978; Scribner and Cole, 1979; Solassol *et al.*, 1979; Strobel *et al.*, 1978; Wahren *et al.*, 1973).

Indications

In this chapter, we deal with our experience in the parenteral nutrition of patients suffering from cancer, but the same general principles apply to patients suffering from a variety of other clinical conditions (see Chapter 4).

For inpatients with cancer, parenteral nutrition is frequently employed during the period preceding conventional therapy for cancer and also during the course of chemotherapy or radiotherapy (Solassol *et al.*, 1979). Each day we treat at least 30 cancer patients in our Nutrition Unit of the Anticancer Centre of Montpellier, which is a part of the Department of Surgery. Additional patients are treated in the various other departments of the Centre, amounting to at least another 30 patients every day.

For outpatients, ambulatory parenteral nutrition is carried out at home. During the period 1972–1979, 58 patients were placed on home parenteral nutrition. There were various reasons for employing this form of nutrition (Table 7.1). The number of patients greatly increased during 1979 because of the systematic use of disposable nutritive bags made of Ethyl-Vinyl-Acetate (E.V.A.). In January 1980 we had 12 patients on home parenteral nutrition.

Home parenteral nutrition technique

Since 1972 we have used the following techniques in our Nutrition Unit (Joyeux and Astruc, 1980). For short-term nutrition, the infusion is given into a superficial vein, for average-term nutrition we employ catheterization of a deep vein (internal jugular or external iliac), and for long-term nutrition we catheterize a collateral of a deep vein. In all cases, only normonutrition mixtures are used (glucose concentration of the mixture less than 15% and total osmolarity of the mixture less than or equal to 1000).

The various techniques are used according to the indications for parenteral nutrition and the precise duration judged to be necessary for each patient (Table 7.2).

Mode of application of home nutrition

Three types of regimen are used. Partial parenteral nutrition is used at

Table 7.1. *Indications for home parenteral feeding in our patients with cancer*

Diagnosis and Treatment	Number of Patients
Ulcerative colitis with cancer (pre-operative)	1
Total bowel resection or obstruction by cancer	6
Gangrenous enteritis after surgery for cancer of the digestive tract	2
Intestinal infarction in cancer patients	3
Post-operative complications fistulas	4
Sequelae or radiation for Hodgkin's disease	6
Sequelae of pelvic radiation	8
Sequelae of abdomino-pelvic radiation	7
Sequelae of total gastrectomy	2
Sequential chemotherapy	19
Total	58

        H. Joyeux and Cl. Solassol

Table 7.2. *Different types of vascular access*

	Superficial Veins	Silicone Catheter	Cannula
Rectocolitis with cancer	–	1	–
Total bowel resection	–	2	4
Gangrenous enteritis	–	2	–
Intestinal infarction	–	1	2
Post-operative fistulas	–	2	2
Sequelae or radiotherapy for Hodgkin's disease	–	3	3
Sequelae of pelvic radiation	1	7	1
Sequelae of abdomino-pelvic radiotherapy	2	5	2
Sequelae of total gastrectomy	–	2	–
Sequential chemotherapy	6	13	6
Total	9	38	20

home when the patient is able to take some food by mouth. Total parenteral nutrition is given when the patient cannot eat. Sequential parenteral nutrition is used for one week per month in patients receiving sequential chemotherapy.

Except for the ten patients first perfused by the superficial venous route, in whom the vascular access was changed on average every three days, the same vascular access has been used throughout the whole period of artificial nutrition.

Patient education

The preparation of patients for home nutrition is carried out during their hospital stay by a team of specialized nurses who are responsible for the theoretical and practical education of the patient. This process is completed within one week. With some patients, we prefer to entrust the practical details of the home parenteral nutrition to the patient's private nurse or to a member of his family.

Outpatient management

All patients placed on home parenteral nutrition receive normonutrition nutritive mixtures prepared by the Pharmacy of our Institute. These mixtures are stored under refrigeration at home for a period lasting from one week to 15 days. The dressings around the catheters are changed once a week by the patient or his nurse. Patient surveillance is carried out once a week by the treating physician, who checks the patient's temperature chart and, if necessary, draws up a balance chart of the patient's serum and urinary electrolytes. The balance chart is drawn up systematically at least twice a month at the time of outpatient attendances. Values for total plasma, protein, albumin, SGOT, SGPT, alkaline phosphatase and serum iron are obtained for all patients on each outpatient visit.

Parenteral nutrition formulae are adapted in accordance with the needs of the patient.

Results

The patients were carefully selected by the Surgery and Nutrition teams, always avoiding the utilization of parenteral nutrition as a method for needlessly prolonging survival in hopeless clinical situations.

Clinical benefits

In all cases, total parenteral nutrition, sequential or continuous, permitted the maintenance or amelioration of the nutritional status of the patient obtained during the hospitalization period of artificial nutrition.

Treatment of malnutrition

All these patients had been or were being treated for a cancer at the outset of parenteral nutrition.

A detailed review of the clinical histories shows that 15 patients suffered from sequelae of cancer treatment. Parenteral nutrition in the hospital and then at home brought about a satisfactory nutritional state.

**Parenteral nutrition as a therapeutic adjuvant
of oncological treatment**

In 27 patients, parenteral nutrition was used in association with specific
treatment of the cancer. This specific treatment was performed at home
(chemotherapy), on an outpatient basis (radiotherapy) or during
hospitalization (surgery), before or after the period of home artificial
nutrition.

Parenteral nutrition as definitive nutritional support

Home parenteral nutrition was carried out in 16 patients with metastatic
cancers, in whom nutritional support was essential for the patient's survival. Four of these patients died, one as a result of myocardial infarction
on the 97th day of home parenteral nutrition, the second of metabolic
dysfunction due to an inoperable obstruction on the 68th day, the
third from diffuse hepatic insufficiency on the 62nd day, and the fourth
from widespread bony metastases.

Complications

Nutritional and metabolic equilibrium failed to be maintained in the
patients of this series who died during treatment. Progressive hepatic
insufficiency with hypoalbuminaemia and ascites appeared in one case
and a metabolic alkalosis with progressive renal insufficiency was
observed in another. No metabolic disorder occurred in the case of the
patient who died of myocardial infarction, nor in another who had to
be given strong analgesics to combat pain.

Nutritional deficiencies were observed in five patients. Dermatitis
secondary to an essential fatty acid deficiency was observed twice in
one patient when she received no lipids, after one month on the first
occasion and after 15 days on the second. Three patients developed
neurological symptoms with nystagmus, which regressed after the
intensive administration of vitamin B_1 by the intramuscular route
(200 mg per day). Another patient developed parasthesiae, described as
'burning of the soles of the feet', which disappeared after the administration of pantothenic acid (500 mg per day) and the other associated
B vitamins.

Technical complications

The objective was to maintain the same vascular access throughout the period of home nutrition. This objective was attained in 50 patients, although a few of these temporarily received parenteral nutrition by superficial veins. In all, 67 vascular accesses were used in 57 patients. One patient, a young woman with two children, was unusual in requiring 13 vascular accesses over the course of 1,927 days of parenteral nutrition. She was psychologically very unstable and reluctant to admit the necessity for parenteral feeding. One cannula remained in place for seven months and another for six months, but the other cannulae had to be withdrawn, either because of obstruction caused by non-rinsing by the patient or because of infectious causes related to the patient herself.

Infectious complications

These complications are certainly the most dangerous. They appeared in three patients and a germ (enterococcus) was isolated after culture of the catheter in one patient out of 57, a rate of infectious complications of 1·4%. In the young married woman mentioned above, four germs were successively isolated, an enterococcus, *Staphylococcus aureus, Streptococcus faecalis* and *Escherichia coli.*

In no case did the infection lead to septicaemia.

Discussion

Home parenteral feeding fills an important place in the therapeutic arsenal in oncology. Nutritional support has become an important therapeutic adjuvant which renders possible oncological treatments that might otherwise be impossible or interrupted. It is a therapeutic measure easily accepted by patients because it is non-aggressive and is not un-comfortable.

This type of parenteral nutrition can be considered after 15 days of hospital nutrition in patients who can then have parenteral nutrition at home for time periods exceeding one month. Apart from patients with terminal cancer, ambulatory and home parenteral nutrition can be carried out in all patients with cancer during anti-neoplasia treatment or at the stage of sequelae. The restoration of nutritional equilibrium will often allow the patient to regain normal digestive function with or without the addition of another treatment.

The level of metabolic and infectious complications is no greater when parenteral nutrition is carried out at home than when it is used in hospital. The rate is very low provided the patient has a good standard of cleanliness and a proper understanding of the basic principles of rigorous asepsis.

This type of nutrition deserves to be more widely used as it leads to a reduction in the duration of hospital stay and thus in the cost of treatment. The value of home parenteral feeding is likely to become comparable to that already observed for home dialysis during the past ten years. As Dudrick remarked recently 'I think in a country that can afford a billion-dollar home dialysis program, we can certainly afford some kind of catastrophic care for patients who through a quirk of fate lose all, or most of their gastrointestinal tract; because these people, after all, are able to work and function and have excellent mentation. They just can't eat.' (Dudrick *et al.*, 1979).

References

Byrne W.J., Burke M., Fonkalsrud F.W. and Anent M.E. (1979) *J. Parent. Ent. Nutr.* 5, 355.

Dudrick S.J., Engelert D.M., Van Buren C.T., Bowland B.J. and MacFayden B.V. (1979) *J. Parent. Ent. Nutr.* 3, 72.

Enger S.C., Herbjornsen K., Eriksson J. and Fretland A. (1977) *Scand. J. chir. lab. Invest.* 37, 252.

Felig P. and Wahren J. (1971) *J. clin. Invest.* 50, 2703.

Heizer W.D. and Orringer E.P. (1977) *Gastroenterology*, 72, 527.

Jeejeebhoy K.N., Langer B., Tsallas G. *et al.* (1976) *Gastroenterology*, 71, 943.

Joyeux H. and Astruc B. (1980) *Traité de Nutrition Artificielle*, Vol. I. Société Scientifique du Traité de Nutrition Artificielle.

Miller D.G. and Ivey M.F. (1979) *J. Parent. Ent. Nutr.* 6, 457.

Powell-Tuck J., Farwell J.A., Nielsen T. and Lennard-Jones J.E. (1978) *Lancet,* ii, 825.

Scribner B.H. and Cole J.J. (1979) *J. Parent. Ent. Nutr.* 2, 58.

Solassol Cl., Joyeux H. and Dubois J.B. (1979) *Nutr. Cancer,* 3, 13.

Strobel C.T., Byrne W.J., Fonkalsrud E.W. and Ament M.E. (1978) *Ann. Surg.* 3, 394.

Wahren J., Felig P., Hendler R. and Ahlborg G. (1973) *J. Appl. Physiol.* 34, 838.

Treatment of Crohn's Disease

Chapter 8
An overall view

J. E. LENNARD-JONES

Improved diagnostic techniques, especially radiology, endoscopy and biopsy, now enable Crohn's disease to be diagnosed in the absence of severe structural changes in the gut. Diagnosis is thus possible in some patients at a stage when the inflammation is potentially reversible without severe disorganisation of structure.

The disease can affect any part of the gut from the mouth to the anus. Even when the inflammation is apparently localised to one segment of the intestine, quantitative histological techniques show that changes are present in apparently normal areas, and sensitive radiological methods and multiple biopsies may show unsuspected and symptomless lesions of Crohn's disease at a distance from the main lesion.

At various times a patient with Crohn's disease may benefit from drug therapy, surgical treatment or nutritional support. The results of several controlled trials now enable some guidelines on drug therapy to be suggested. Surgical treatment is needed for most patients at some stage, and usually involves removal of a severely affected part of the gut. The widespread nature of the disease is probably the reason why recurrent inflammation develops over ten or more years in about half the patients treated by resection and anastomosis. There is some debate as to whether or not dietary manipulation affects inflammation; there is no doubt that many patients need replacement of nutritional deficits.

Surgical treatment

Clear indications for operation are the structural complications (Fig.

8.1) of perforation, abscess formation, obstruction, entero-cutaneous or internal fistulae, peri-anal fistulae or gynaecological complications. In general, a chronic entero-cutaneous fistula associated with an abscess does not heal unless the underlying diseased intestine from which it arises is resected. Persistent severe inflammation of the gut unresponsive to drug therapy in acceptable doses is often treated surgically provided that it is technically possible to remove or bypass the diseased segment.

The relative merits of resection or bypass seem to have been settled in favour of resection whenever possible. There is still some controversy about the extent of resection; a possible reduced or delayed recurrence rate after wide resection of apparently normal intestine on either side of a lesion has to be balanced against the nutritional and symptomatic consequences of removal of functional intestine. A trend towards conservation of grossly normal intestine is apparent. A policy of restricting surgical treatment to severely diseased segments, without attempted extirpation of all diseased areas, is acceptable when Crohn's disease is widespread.

STRUCTURAL COMPLICATIONS

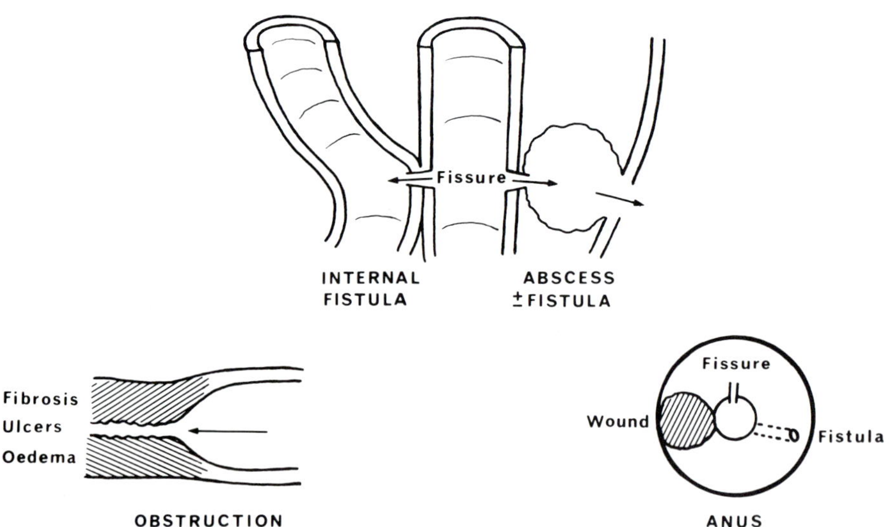

Fig. 8.1. *Some structural complications.*

The role of diversion operations, such as the split ileostomy is debatable; most centres prefer immediate resection and anastomosis without a preliminary phase of diversion. Since the recurrence rate at a stoma is usually less than at an anastomosis, there has been a tendency to favour proctocolectomy and ileostomy for Crohn's colitis, even when the rectum is only slightly diseased. Even though inflammation often does develop in the region of the anastomosis, many patients continue to feel well and their symptoms can be controlled by drugs. The success of this and other operations should be gauged by the satisfaction of the patient rather than by pathological findings.

Nutritional aspects of treatment

Diet as a primary treatment

There is epidemiological evidence that patients with Crohn's disease eat more sugar, and less raw fruit and vegetables, than other people. One retrospective study, using matched controls treated in other clinics, has suggested that an unrefined-carbohydrate, fibre-rich diet is beneficial in that time spent in hospital and the number of operations was less among those who took this diet than among those who had no dietary instruction (Heaton *et al.*, 1979). A prospective controlled trial of this diet is now being undertaken.

Other workers have recommended as a primary treatment the use of a chemically-defined diet, or parenteral nutrition, with the aim of eliminating food from the lumen of the diseased intestine. So far, these claims are unsupported by controlled data, and the concept of 'bowel rest' as a treatment awaits proof.

Diet for relief of symptoms

In patients with multiple strictures not amenable to surgical treatment, a liquid or semi-solid diet may relieve bolus colic.

Patients suffering from diarrhoea due to steatorrhoea may be helped by a low fat diet. Those with diarrhoea due to lactose intolerance are benefited by milk restriction.

Restoration of lost tissue, growth and prevention of specific deficiencies

ASSESSMENT OF DEFICIENCIES

Every patient's nutritional state should be assessed in terms of weight, height and specific haematological and biochemical deficits. The weight of adults should be expressed as a proportion of the usual (or optimal) value. During childhood and adolescence, weight and height should be plotted on a percentile chart so that both can be expressed in terms of the normal range for the same age and sex. Whenever possible, the growth rate should be determined by plotting measurements recorded in the past and at every follow-up visit. Simple skin fold and arm circumference measurements can add to the basic data by providing information on body fat content, lean body mass and muscle bulk.

WHY HAVE DEFICIENCIES DEVELOPED?

Dietary intake can be simply and quickly assessed by recording a typical day's meals. If relevant, this description should be supplemented by a formal assessment so that the daily intake of energy and protein is expressed quantitatively. This simple measure often shows that the patient is taking less than the 30–35 Cal/kg needed to maintain weight, not to say regain weight or grow, while undertaking some activity and allowing for the effects of inflammation. Further enquiry will reveal whether the reduced food intake is due to the poor appetite of systemic illness, the nausea and sense of fullness of chronic obstruction, or a wish to reduce bolus colic and/or diarrhoea.

Malabsorption contributes to specific deficiencies, such as vitamin B_{12}, but little to deficits of energy and protein even though malabsorption of fat is demonstrable by chemical measurement. *Losses,* especially of protein, may be considerable from areas of severe mucosal inflammation. The depressing effect of *chronic inflammation* on blood formation, and probably on protein synthesis, must be recognised. For example, the apparent iron deficiency anaemia of chronic disease with normal marrow iron stores, low serum iron and low total iron binding capacity is a common finding.

Treatment

Treatment of the *primary disease* may make a major contribution to nutrition by relief of symptoms, increased appetite, decreased losses and improved synthesis.

A daily *energy requirement* of 2,500 or 3,000 Cal (10·5 or 12·6MJ) may sometimes be difficult to meet. The patient must be encouraged to take adequate sized meals of appropriate food with frequent snacks in between. Liquid supplements, usually based on milk (e.g. 'Complan', 'Build-up' etc.) may be used as snacks but should not be given in such a way that appetite is reduced.

For some patients a supplemental feed given at night slowly and continuously through a very fine nasogastric tube enables about 1,000 Cal (4·2MJ) to be added to the daily intake. For other patients a tube feed giving 3,000 Cals (12·6MJ) over 24 hours is needed. Parenteral nutrition is indicated for the patient with obstruction, a high entero-cutaneous fistula or a very short small intestine.

Vitamin B_{12}, for all patients who have lost more than 100 cm of distal ileum, folic acid and/or iron, are commonly needed. Patients with severe fluid losses may need magnesium and zinc, those with severe fat malabsorption may need Vitamins D and K.

'Short gut syndrome'

A few patients are left with a very short length of jejunum anastomosed to colon or ending at a stoma. Losses of intestinal secretions may amount to 3 or more litres of fluid daily, containing about 100 mmol of sodium per litre. Some water taken by mouth is absorbed but the remainder increases fluid output and increases sodium loss. Conservation of sodium is the major therapeutic problem in these patients. Absorption of sodium taken by mouth can be increased by giving it with glucose, or better a glucose polymer such as starch or 'caloreen' (Griffin *et al.*, 1980). Water and salt can be further conserved by codeine phosphate, loperamide and/or diphenoxylate in full doses and sometimes in combination.

Occasionally the remaining healthy intestine is inadequate to maintain nutrition and fluid balance. In such patients parenteral nutrition, self administered as a long-term treatment at home, offers the only chance of health. Some of these patients find it better to take a little or nothing by mouth, others use the parenteral feed as a supplement to a reduced oral intake.

Drug therapy

Drugs used in the treatment of Crohn's disease may be broadly grouped
into anti-inflammatory drugs, drugs that may affect immune responses,
anti-bacterial drugs and symptomatic treatments. Some of the drugs
have been shown by controlled trial to give benefit in particular circumstances, but not in others. Other drugs have been tested but no benefit
has been demonstrable within the conditions of the trial; these trials are
mentioned for completeness. Certain drugs have not yet been subjected
to controlled trial but anecdotal reports encourage further study of
their use.

Anti-inflammatory drugs

Sulphasalazine

This drug, salicyl-azo-sulphapyridine (Fig. 8.2) is split at the azo link by
enteric bacteria to yield 5-aminosalicylic acid and sulphapyridine. The
former is largely excreted in the stool whereas the sulphapyridine is
almost completely absorbed and is then excreted in the urine after

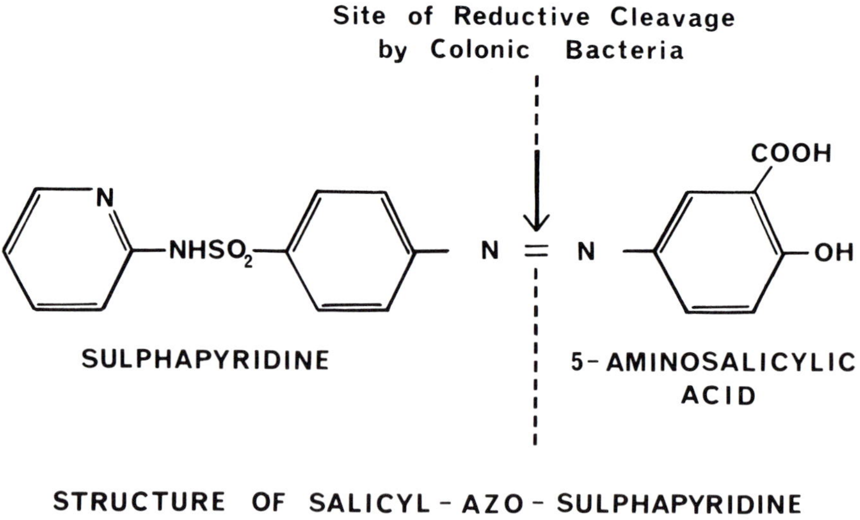

Fig. 8.2. *The structure of sulphasalazine showing the site of cleavage by
enteric bacteria.*

conjugation. Observations in ulcerative colitis suggest that the 5-amino-salicylic acid is the active moiety and it is possible that the parent molecule acts as a carrier which liberates 5-aminosalicylic acid when enteric bacteria are encountered in the intestinal lumen.

THERAPEUTIC TRIALS (TABLE 8.1)

(a) Active disease : Sulphasalazine, 1 g/15 kg body weight (maximum 5 g) daily, proved no better than placebo in ileal disease, but was effective in ileo-colic ($P = 0.027$) and colonic disease ($P = 0.006$) (Summers *et al.*, 1979). Analysis of data in another smaller trial (Anthonisen *et al.*, 1974) also shows no certain benefit in disease confined to the small bowel but a therapeutic effect in ileo-colic and colonic disease ($P = < 0.05$). (The authors' analysis demonstrates benefit in patients treated without previous surgical treatment, but not in patients after resection. From their data in Tables 8.1, 8.2 and 8.4 it is also possible to analyse

Table 8.1. *Controlled trials of sulphasalazine*

Type of disease	Control	Patients Sulphasalazine	Result	P	Reference
'Active'					
Ileum	25	17			Summers *et al.*, 1979
Ileo-colic	43	49	+	0·027	Summers *et al.*, 1979
Colon	9	8	+	0·006	Summers *et al.*, 1979
Ileum*	11X		−		Anthonisen *et al.*, 1974
Ileo-colic/ colon	14X		+	<0·05	Anthonisen *et al.*, 1974
'Inactive'	88	43	−		Summers *et al.*, 1979
After Resection	35	49**	−		Bergman and Krause, 1976
	19	14	−		Multicentre, 1977
	34	32	−		Wenckert *et al.*, 1978
	13	15	−		Summers *et al.*, 1979

*See text.
**Sulphasalazine and prednisolone given in reducing doses over 33 weeks.

the results according to the site of disease and to test their significance with Wilcoxon's 2-tail rank sum test).

(b) Inactive disease: A trial over 1–2 years among patients with inactive disease failed to show that sulphasalazine in a dose of 0·5 g per 15 kg body weight (maximum 2·5 g) daily reduced the relapse rate (Summers *et al.*, 1979).

(c) After resection: Four trials have failed to show that sulphasalazine given over periods of up to 2 years reduces the relapse rate after resection (Bergman and Krause, 1976; Multicentre trial, 1977; Wenckert *et al.*, 1978; Summers *et al.*, 1979).

COMMENT

In practice, sulphasalazine often seems most helpful in patients with a short history of ileo-colitis or Crohn's colitis. Sometimes the drug does appear to be effective in extensive small bowel disease, perhaps because the enteric flora extends proximally in such patients.

At present there are no controlled data to support the use of sulphasalazine in quiescent disease or after resection with the aim of reducing the relapse rate. The authors of one trial (Wenckert *et al.*, 1978) calculate that 110–130 patients would be needed in each treatment group to ensure a high probability of showing that the relapse rate is halved by treatment. Until a trial of this size is completed the effectiveness of sulphasalazine as a maintenance treatment remains unproven but results are not encouraging.

Interest must centre on the development of analogues of sulphasalazine and studies on its mode of action. Would 5-amino salicylic acid given by mouth be helpful in extensive small bowel disease? Can a carrier molecule with less potential toxicity than sulphapyridine be found to deliver 5-amino salicylic acid to the distal ileum and colon? Does sulphapyridine contribute to the therapeutic effectiveness of the drug?

Corticosteroids (Table 8.2)

THERAPEUTIC TRIALS

(a) Active disease: A multicentre trial (Summers *et al.*, 1979) has shown that prednisone 0·25–0·75 mg/kg body weight (maximum 60 mg) daily, the dose being adjusted to the activity of the disease, was more effective than placebo ($P < 0.0006$). These results applied to patients with ileal ($P = 0.002$) and ileo-colic disease ($P = 0.008$), but the results in patients with colonic disease were not significant, perhaps due to the small size of the group.

(b) Inactive disease/After resection: Three trials have failed to show benefit from low doses of corticosteroids in preventing relapse in patients with inactive disease after medical treatment or after resection. Prednisone, 7·5 mg daily for up to 3 years, did not improve the relapse rate nor did it affect recurrence or extension of disease among 33 patients compared with 26 patients receiving a control tablet (Smith *et al.*, 1978). Prednisone, 0·25 mg/kg body weight (max. 20 mg) daily was not apparently superior to placebo over 1–2 years in maintaining remission (Summers *et al.*, 1979). Prednisolone, reducing from 15 to 5 mg daily over 33 weeks after resection (with sulphasalazine 3 g daily) and then stopping treatment, failed to reduce the recurrence rate over the first 3 post-operative years (Bergman and Krause, 1976).

COMMENT

Corticosteroids given in adequate doses (20–60 mg daily) often control acute exacerbations of the disease. Clinical experience, and the difficulty experienced in several trials of weaning patients from smaller doses, suggest that the drugs given in the long-term can suppress activity in chronic disease. Further studies are needed on long-term corticosteroid treatment. Is there a minimal effective dose and does this vary from patient to patient? Is a double dose of a corticosteroid drug given in the morning on alternate days as effective, but with fewer side effects, as half that dose given every day?

Whenever possible, corticosteroids should be given in an adequate dose for a short period and then withdrawn. Long-term corticosteroid therapy should be used only when safer drugs such as sulphasalazine are ineffective and when it has been shown that withdrawal of the corticosteroid leads to relapse. In such patients the possible need for surgical treatment or long-term azathioprine should be considered so that corticosteroids can be reduced or stopped.

Combination of a corticosteroid and sulphasalazine

Since both drugs are effective in the treatment of many patients with active Crohn's disease, it is reasonable to test whether or not the

 J. E. Lennard-Jones

Table 8.2. *Controlled trials of corticosteroid drugs*

Type of disease and daily dose	Patients		Result	*P*	Reference
	Control	*Prednis(ol)one*			
'Active'					
0·25—0·75 mg/kg	77	85	+	<0·0006	Summers *et al.*, 1979
'Inactive' or after resection					
7·5 mg	26	33	—		Smith *et al.*, 1978
15 → 5 mg	35	49	—		Bergman and Krause, 1976
0·25 mg/kg	101	61	—		Summers *et al.*, 1979

Table 8.3. *Controlled trials of azathioprine*

Type of disease and daily dose	Patients		Result	*P*	Reference
	Control	*Azathioprine*			
'Active'					
2 mg/kg		15X	—		Rhodes *et al.*, 1971
3 mg/kg		27X	—		Klein *et al.*, 1974
2·5 mg/kg	77	59			Summers *et al.*, 1979
'Maintenance'					
2 mg/kg	11	11	+	<0·01	Willoughby *et al.*, 1971
2 mg/kg	10	10	+	<0·05	Rosenberg *et al.*, 1975
2 mg/kg	27	24	+	<0·01	O'Donoghue *et al.*, 1978
1 mg/kg	101	54	—		Summers *et al.*, 1979

beneficial effects are additive. In fact, a controlled trial of prednisone, with or without sulphasalazine, has failed to show that the addition of sulphasalazine increased the rate of remission in active disease, reduced the relapse rate in patients with inactive disease, or that sulphasalazine exerted a steroid-sparing effect (Singleton *et al.*, 1979). A combination of sulphasalazine and prednisolone given in reducing doses over 33 weeks after resection failed to influence the relapse rate over the next 3 years (Bergman and Krause, 1976).

Agents with a possible effect on immunity

Two drugs, azathioprine and 6-mercaptopurine, could affect Crohn's disease by depressing immune responses, although the drugs also have anti-inflammatory and perhaps other properties. Disodium cromoglycate has been tested for its possible stabilising effect on intestinal mast cells. Several agents have been given with the aim of stimulating cellular immunity but without demonstrable benefit.

Azathioprine (Table 8.3)

THERAPEUTIC TRIALS

(a) Active disease: Three trials have failed to show that azathioprine 2–3 mg/kg body weight daily is an effective treatment for active Crohn's disease. Two trials (Rhodes *et al.*, 1971; Klein *et al.*, 1974) were of cross-over design with trial periods of 2 and 4 months; the third (Summers *et al.*, 1979) was a comparison between two treatment groups over 4 months.

(b) Maintenance treatment: Azathioprine, 2 mg/kg body weight daily, has been shown to maintain control of quiescent or chronically active disease. The first trial (Willoughby *et al.*, 1971) assessed the effect of giving azathioprine or a control tablet with prednisolone, which was withdrawn once the disease was quiescent. Ten of 11 patients on azathioprine remained in remission, whereas 8 of 11 on placebo relapsed ($P<0.01$). Another trial (Rosenberg *et al.*, 1975) assessed the ability to reduce a maintenance dose of prednisone of at least 10 mg daily in a group of 10 patients given azathioprine as compared with a similar group given a control tablet. The mean reduction in the prednisone dose among the group given azathioprine was greater ($P<0.05$)

than in the control group; relapses tended to be commoner in the latter. The most recent trial (O'Donoghue *et al.*, 1978) tested the effect of withdrawing azathioprine under double blind conditions from a group of 27 patients who had been treated with the drug for more than 6 months and who were in good health. Nine patients relapsed compared with one relapse among the control group of 24 patients who continued azathioprine ($P < 0.01$). It was not possible to correlate the relapse rate with the duration of previous remission or of azathioprine treatment. The only trial that has failed to show benefit from azathioprine as a maintenance treatment (Summers *et al.*, 1979) used a dose of 1 mg/kg body weight daily.

COMMENT

Azathioprine appears to be a useful drug for maintaining remission after corticosteroid treatment of an acute attack and for controlling the inflammation in patients with chronic active disease, sometimes in combination with other drugs. As in other disorders it has a steroid-sparing effect. Clinical observation suggests that it has a slow action, perhaps over months. The failure of the trials in acute disease may have been because they were relatively short and because azathioprine was given alone.

Azathioprine is potentially dangerous and one patient in the published trials died of marrow suppression (O'Donoghue *et al.*, 1978). Other patients had to discontinue the drug becase of acute pancreatitis, leucopenia, dyspepsia or fever (Summers *et al.*, 1979). The drug should not be used in a dose greater than 2·5 mg/kg body weight and regular haemoglobin, white cell and platelet measurements should be closely supervised. Azathioprine should be reserved for patients with severe Crohn's disease whose symptoms are due to inflammation rather than structural complications of the disease and in whom the potential hazards are justified. Unfortunately, it is not possible at present to define the duration of maintenance therapy but the withdrawal trial quoted showed relapses in patients who had been treated continuously for more than 2 years.

6-Mercaptopurine

TRIAL

A double-blind cross-over study among 83 patients with chronic Crohn's disease, unresponsive to other drugs in which 6-mercaptopurine 1·5 mg/ kg body weight daily, or a placebo, were added to existing treatment, showed more frequent ($P<0.0001$) improvement in the active group (Present *et al.*, 1980). The therapeutic response could occur several months after starting treatment. There was no mortality but about 10% of patients developed severe side-effects including marrow depression, febrile reaction, pancreatitis and nausea.

COMMENT

Azathioprine is a derivative of 6-mercaptopurine and it seems likely that the two drugs can be used in a similar way.

Other drugs given with the aim of affecting immune response

Levamisole (Wesdorp *et al.*, 1977; Swarbrick and O'Donoghue, 1979), oral BCG (Burnham *et al.*, 1979), transfer factor (Vicary *et al.*, 1979) and disodium cromoglycate (Grundman *et al.*, 1978) have been tested in controlled trials without demonstrable benefit.

Anti-bacterial drugs

Anti-bacterial drugs may affect secondary infection or reduce the antigenic stimulus of enteric bacteria. An uncontrolled study has suggested that broad spectrum antibiotics given continuously in various combinations over periods of up to 5 years can result in considerable benefit (Moss *et al.*, 1978). The only anti-bacterial drug tested so far by controlled trial is metronidazole.

Metronidazole

This drug is bactericidal to anaerobic bacteria but it does not appear to affect the intestinal flora greatly unless given with another drug effective against aerobes.

THERAPEUTIC TRIAL

In a small double-blind cross-over trial (Blichfeldt *et al.*, 1978) among

20 patients given metronidazole 1 g daily for 2 months in addition to other treatments, clinical and haematological improvement ($P<0.01$) was noted among the 6 patients with colonic disease, but among the group as a whole the only significant effects were a rise in the haemoglobin level and a fall in the sedimentation rate during the metronidazole period.

COMMENT

Other uncontrolled observations have also suggested that metronidazole may be most effective among patients with colonic and ano-rectal disease, although the controlled study was disappointing. Combination of metronidazole with a drug bactericidal to aerobic organisms, such as co-trimoxazole or an aminoglycoside, seems logical and clinical results often seem to justify the temporary use of such a combination of anti-bacterial drugs. Metronidazole can cause paraesthesiae, hallucinations, headache and alcohol intolerance so it should be used with care.

Other antibacterial drugs

Dapsone apparently benefited 4 of 6 patients to whom it was given (Ward and McManus, 1975). Anti-tuberculous therapy, before the introduction of rifampicin and other newer drugs, did not appear beneficial.

Symptomatic drug treatment

Anti-diarrhoeal drugs

Double-blind cross-over studies have shown that loperamide decreases stool frequency and weight, with a corresponding trend towards solid consistency in Crohn's disease, or after ileo-colic resection, or after colectomy and ileo-rectal anastomosis (Pelemans and Vantrappen, 1976; Mainguet and Fiasse, 1977). In the first of these trials, loperamide at a mean dose of 6·9 mg daily was shown to be superior to diphenoxylate, at a mean dose of 17·7 mg daily, in terms of stool frequency and consistency ($P = 0.01$) and patients' preference ($P = 0.002$). Loperamide (Tytgat and Huibregtse, 1975) and codeine phosphate (Newton,

1978) both reduce ileostomy output by about 20–25%, whereas diphenoxylate appears to be less effective.

When the terminal ileum is diseased or after ileal resection, bile salts entering the colon may cause secretion of water and electrolytes, and thus diarrhoea. Cholestyramine, 4g with meals or sometimes in smaller doses, may be helpful in this situation.

Anti-spasmodic and analgesic drugs

Anti-spasmodics are of doubtful benefit. Certain patients with chronic pain, unrelieved by measures already outlined, seem to need regular doses of non-addictive analgesic drugs.

Treatment of different types of Crohn's disease

Extensive small bowel disease

There may be extensive mucosal inflammation or multiple short segments of disease. Surgical treatment is generally limited to resection or bypass of short segments which cause obstruction. Some patients with pain and/or malabsorption respond well to corticosteroids, perhaps with a low-residue or low-fat diet. Azathioprine may be needed for such patients to enable remission to be maintained and the corticosteroid dose to be reduced or stopped. Sulphasalazine is not usually effective. Short courses of anti-bacterial drugs may apparently benefit acute exacerbations. Some patients remain well and symptom-free without drug treatment, despite severe radiological changes.

Terminal ileal and ileo-colic disease

Patients with this form of disease tend to develop obstructive symptoms or abscess formation. Surgical treatment is often needed and resection is usually possible. Since operation is often followed by long or apparently permanent relief of symptoms, particularly if the diseased segment is short, surgical treatment has much to commend it. Drug treatment can include sulphasalazine, corticosteroids and anti-bacterial drugs. Unfortunately, no long-term drug treatment has yet been found which reduces the recurrence rate after resection.

                    J. E. Lennard-Jones

Crohn's colitis

Acute attacks of this form of colitis behave and respond very similarly to acute attacks of ulcerative colitis. Urgent surgical treatment may be needed for perforation, colonic dilatation or failure to respond to drug therapy. Prednisolone, 60 mg daily, intravenously may be needed for the severe attack. Prednisolone by mouth, or by retention enema, can be used in less severe attacks. Sulphasalazine alone is a useful treatment for mild attacks. Antibacterial drugs, including metronidazole, may be helpful. Azathioprine may be used for chronic disease which fails to respond to other drugs, especially when corticosteroids cannot be withdrawn without relapse. Surgical treatment, usually colectomy with ileostomy or ileo-rectal anastomosis, may be needed for chronic disease or complications.

Ano-rectal disease

Although severe lesions may cause gross structural changes, symptoms can be slight. Abscesses require surgical drainage and superficial fistulae can be laid open. Complex fistulae are best treated with a conservative surgical approach limited to the provision of free drainage and designed to conserve the sphincter. Complex lesions may heal or become symptomless if the intestinal disease becomes quiescent. Antibacterial drugs, including metronidazole, can benefit acute infective episodes.

Residual or recurrent disease after surgical treatment

Recurrent disease at an anastomosis or stoma can be treated as already described. Large unhealed anal or perianal wounds, sometimes associated with ulceration in the groins and natal cleft, which fail to heal with meticulous nursing care, sometimes seem to respond to corticosteroids and azathioprine.

General principles

An over-simplified, but perhaps helpful, concept of different types of disease is shown in Figure 8.3. *Mucosal disease* may cause diarrhoea, pain, malabsorption, or exudation with losses of blood and protein. The inflammatory response may cause systemic symptoms, growth

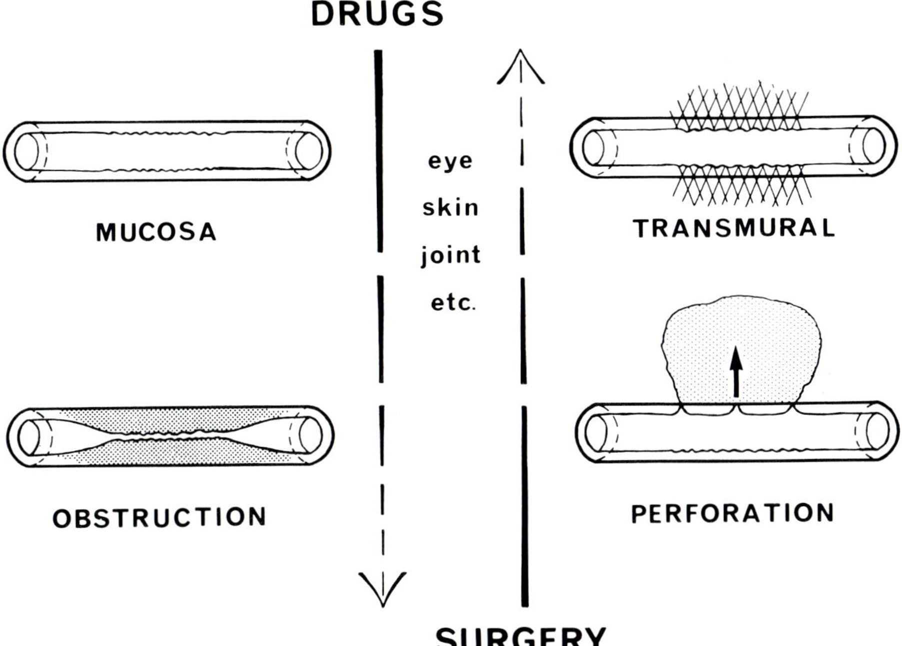

Fig. 8.3. *The relative importance of medical and surgical treatments in different types of disease.*

failure, the anaemia of chronic disease, and associated lesions such as erythema nodosum, arthritis or iritis. This type of disease is usually helped by corticosteroids, and often by sulphasalazine, especially if the distal ileum and/or colon are involved. Azathioprine may be beneficial in the long term once acute symptoms have improved.

Transmural inflammation leads to local tenderness and thickening of the gut wall, with possible involvement of related structures in addition to the features already described. Secondary infection may be an important factor. Antibacterial drugs, perhaps combined with an anti-inflammatory drug, may be appropriate.

Surgical treatment may be needed for mucosal or transmural disease if there is no improvement with drug therapy and resection of the diseased area is practicable. Surgical treatment is more often needed for the *structural complications* of obstruction, perforation, abscess or fistula formation. In these situation drugs have a limited role. Corticosteroids can lead to improvement of obstructive symptoms, presumably due to reduction of local oedema and swelling of the gut wall,

                  J. E. Lennard-Jones

but surgical treatment is generally required later. Antibacterial drugs have a limited role in the control of infection at the time of operation and of chronic infective lesions.

Nutritional and symptomatic treatments may be needed in all types of Crohn's disease and are an important aspect of management.

Crohn's disease is often a long-term debilitating illness. Support and encouragement of the patient and his family, preferably with continuity of clinical care over many years, and flexibility in the use of different types of treatment appropriate to changing phases of the disease, is the best that we can offer at present.

References

Anthonisen P., Bárány F., Folkenborg O., Holtz A., Jarnum S., Kristensen M., Riis P., Walan A. and Worning H. (1974) *Scand. J. Gastroenterol.* **9**, 549.

Bergman L. and Krause U. (1976) *Scand. J. Gastroenterol.* **11**, 651.

Blichfeldt P., Blomhoff J.P., Myhre E. and Gjone E. (1978) *Scand. J. Gastroenterol.* **13**, 123.

Burnham W.R., Lennard-Jones J.E., Hecketsweiler P., Colin R. and Geffroy Y. (1979) *Gut,* **20**, 229.

Griffin G., Hodgson H. and Chadwick V.S. (1980) *Clin. Sci.* **58**, 3P.

Grundman M.J., Williams S.E. and Turnberg L.A. (1978) *Gut*, **19**, 963A.

Heaton K.W., Thornton J.R. and Emmett P.M. (1979) *Brit. med. J.* ii, 764.

Klein M., Binder H.J., Mitchell M., Aaronson R. and Spiro H. (1974) *Gastroenterology,* **66**, 916.

Mainguet P. and Fiasse R. (1977) *Gut,* **18**, 575.

Moss A.A., Carbone J.V. and Kressel H.Y. (1978) *Amer. J. Roentgenol.* **131**, 787.

Multicentre Trial (1977) *Gut,* **18**, 69.

Newton C.R. (1968) *Gut,* **19**, 377.

O'Donoghue D.P., Dawson A.M., Powell-Tuck J., Bown R.L. and Lennard-Jones J.E. (1978) *Lancet,* **ii**, 955.

Pelemans W. and Vantrappen G. (1976) *Gastroenterology,* **70**, 1030.

Present D.H., Korelitz B.I., Wisch N., Glass J.L., Sachar D.B. and Pasternack B.S. (1980) *New. Engl. J. Med.* **302**, 981.

Rhodes J., Bainton D., Beck P. and Campbell H. (1971) *Lancet,* **ii**, 1273.

Rosenberg J.L., Levin B., Wall A.J. and Kirsner J.B. (1975) *Amer. J. dig. Dis.* **20**, 721.

Singleton J.W., Summers R.W., Kern F. jr., Becktel J.M., Best W.R., Hansen R.N. and Winship D.H. (1979) *Gastroenterology,* **77**, 887.

Smith R.C., Rhodes J., Heatley R.V., Hughes L.E., Crosby D.L., Rees B.I., Jones H., Evans K.T. and Lawrie B.W. (1978) *Gut,* **19**, 606.

Summers R.W., Switz D.M., Sessions J.T. jr., Becktel J.M., Best W.R., Kern F. jr. and Singleton J.W. (1979) *Gastroenterology,* **77**, 847.

Swarbrick E.T. and O'Donoghue D.P. (1979) *Lancet,* i, 392.

Tytgat G.N. and Huibregtse K. (1975) *Brit. med. J.* ii, 667.

Vicary F.R., Chambers J.D. and Dhillon P. (1979) *Gut,* **20**, 408.

Ward M. and McManus J.P.A. (1975) *Lancet,* **i**, 1236.

Wenckert A., Kristensen M., Eklund A.E., Bárány F., Jarnum S., Worning H., Folkenborg O., Holtz A., Bonnevie O. and Riis P. (1978) *Scand. J. Gastroenterol.* **13**, 161.

Wesdorp E., Schellekens P.T.A., Weening R., Meuwissen S.G.M. and Tytgat G.N.J. (1977) *Gut,* **18**, 971A.

Willoughby J.M.T., Kumar P.J., Beckett J. and Dawson A.M. (1971) *Lancet,* **ii**, 944.

Chapter 9
Nutritional methods

JEREMY POWELL-TUCK

The nutritional treatment of Crohn's disease has two distinct aspects, the first being the treatment of undernutrition and the second being the relief of symptoms or treatment of the disease itself.

The treatment of undernutrition

It is helpful to consider specific nutrient deficiencies, such as vitamin deficiencies, separately from protein energy malnutrition (P.E.M.). However, while specific deficiencies may occur alone, it is unusual for P.E.M. to occur without concomitant specific deficiencies. It is now recognised that improvement or maintenance of body nitrogen mass depends upon the provision not only of adequate calories and protein but also of individual nutrients such as sodium, potassium, phosphorus (Rudman *et al.*, 1975) and zinc (Halsted *et al.*, 1972).

Assessment of nutrition

The nutrition of our patients with Crohn's disease should be routinely assessed. We need to know whether they are eating normally and what their usual weight is. In patients who are obviously thin, we should pay attention to symptoms suggestive of specific deficiencies, such as a sore mouth, aguesia, muscle cramps, paraesthesiae or, rarely, a bruising tendency or night blindness. Nutritional examination should routinely include measurement of weight and a record of height. Measurements of arm circumference and skin fold thickness can prove useful for later comparison. We should note any wasting of muscle or fat, growth impairment, oedema, hepatomegaly and any abnormalities of the skin, nails or hair. There may be anaemia, angular stomatitis, cheilosis or a smooth tongue. More rarely, deficiency syndromes may be manifested by peripheral neuropathy, bruising or tenderness over bones.

Blood tests may reveal anaemia and its cause, the presence of hypo-proteinaemia or electrolyte imbalance, or specific deficiencies. A detailed dietary history, tests of malabsorption and balance studies of energy and protein can then be used to determinate the reasons for the abnormalities.

The prevalence of undernutrition in Crohn's disease

Because the patients attending hospital, either as outpatients or in-patients, are a selected group, we know little of the true prevalence of undernutrition in Crohn's disease. Hill and co-workers (1977) studied 74 patients with inflammatory bowel disease and found that, while those with an ileostomy routinely attending the outpatient clinic were not below weight, 2 out of 15 patients whose disease was in 'remission', 4 out of 12 admitted for elective surgery, 11 out of 22 admitted in an acute attack or for urgent surgery, and 9 out of 9 admitted from other units with post-operative complications weighed less than 90% of their pre-illness weight. The mean weight loss of those coming to urgent surgery was about 10% while it was 25% for those admitted with post-operative complications.

Dyer *et al.* (1972) studied 63 inpatients with Crohn's disease and found that anaemia was present in 40, of whom half had haemoglobin levels below 10 g/100 ml. Anaemia in Crohn's disease is due partly to in-hibition of erythropoiesis by the chronic inflammatory process and partly to depletion of nutrients such as iron, folate and vitamin B_{12}. The prevalence of folate and iron depletion correlated with the pre-valence of active disease in the group studied. They also found that iron stores were absent from the bone marrow in 18 out of 46 patients subjected to marrow aspiration, and that the red cell folate was depleted in 13 out of 37 patients studied. Hoffbrand *et al.* (1968) found the red cell folate to be depleted in 7 out of a subgroup of 19 patients. However, in neither of these papers is it clear to what extent and by what criteria the patients tested were selected from the main group under study. The prevalence of vitamin B_{12} deficiency depends not upon the disease activity but upon the prevalence of terminal ileal resection or disease. Thus, in Dyer's series of 42 patients who had not had a resection, 3 had serum levels of less than 160 pg/ml, while low levels were found in 8 out of 26 patients who had had a resection. Within the resected group, there was a correlation between the level of the serum vitamin B_{12}, the length of time following the surgery and the amount of ileum resected. Levels below 80 pg/ml were associated with resections of 100 cm or more.

Rationale for nutritional treatment

The rationale for treating syndromes attributed to deficiencies of specific nutrients, such as water, electrolytes and vitamins, are so obvious that they require no discussion here. I have also mentioned that specific nutrients may become crucial for the increase or maintenance of the body's mass of nitrogen or other nutrients. Depletion of certain specific nutrients such as zinc or folate can result in depressed cell mediated immunity (Golden, 1978; Gross *et al.*, 1975).

As protein energy malnutrition supervenes, the metabolic rate (Keys *et al.*, 1950), protein turnover (Waterlow *et al.*, 1977) and growth diminish. There is diminished urea and CO_2 production and the heart rate slows (Keys *et al.*, 1950). The decline in the metabolic rate and protein turnover as a response to lack of food appears very quickly, and indeed may be observed between meals in normal subjects. However, at some point in the development of P.E.M., physiological adaptation becomes pathological abnormality. The grossly undernourished patient is weak, apathetic and immobile; he has diminished hypersensitivity reactions, particularly of the delayed type; he is prone to infection and heals his wounds poorly. We do not know at what point this occurs but a study of patients undergoing surgery for peptic ulcer showed that those with a 20% reduction in body weight pre-operatively had an increased likelihood of post-operative complications (Studley, 1936).

Studies have suggested that delayed hypersensitivity and wound healing can be improved by improving nutrition (Law *et al.*, 1973; Steiger *et al.*, 1973). Two controlled trials have suggested that post-operative complications can be reduced by post-operative feeding (Collins *et al.*, 1978; Sagar *et al.*, 1979). A review has suggested that mortality from enterocutaneous fistulas is reduced substantially by nutritional support (Leading Article, *Lancet*, 1979). Thus evidence is accumulating that treatment of P.E.M. in Crohn's disease is likely to be beneficial, particularly in severely ill patients requiring surgery.

Failure of growth is a well recognised adaptation to reduced nutrient intake. In malnourished children, growth is accelerated when ample food is given. Two studies have suggested that growth retardation in Crohn's disease is effectively treated by ensuring adequate nutrient intakes (Layden *et al.*, 1976; Kelts *et al.*, 1979). Intakes in children required for growth are much greater per kilogram body weight than those needed for weight gain in adults (Waterlow, 1978). It remains to be seen, however, whether all the growth retardation which occurs related to Crohn's disease can be corrected nutritionally.

Causes of undernutrition

Before we treat nutrient deficiencies in Crohn's disease, it is helpful to understand how they arise. Undernutrition can be caused by abnormalities of intake, absorption, metabolism and loss. In fact, most deficiencies are caused by several factors operating together, with intake usually the most important.

INTAKE

A careful dietary history will almost always reveal reduced intake in patients undernourished from Crohn's disease. The intake may be diminished due to anorexia, fear of eating, depression or apathy, or because the patient believes that it may be therapeutic to stop eating. Anorexia may be due to the disease itself or to drugs. Fear of eating may arise from a sore mouth, or from fear of abdominal pain, vomiting or diarrhoea. Depression may be related to symptoms, to the sight of fistulae or the presence of a stoma. It may stem from the complicated psychosocial effects of a chronic disease. Apathy may be caused by undernutrition itself and thus may become an important link in a vicious cycle. Far too often in hospital the choice of food offered is unimaginative and the presentation of it poor. Occasionally, changes in taste may play a part and can be due to oral disease, such as candidiasis, the effect of antibiotics, or zinc deficiency.

ABSORPTION

Malabsorption arises for a variety of reasons related to small-intestinal Crohn's disease. The inflamed mucosa may be unable to absorb normally. Stricturing or entero-enteric fistulae may result in blind loops or stagnation of the intestinal contents with bacterial overgrowth. Resections of the specialised terminal ileum may give rise to specific deficiencies and massive resections may result in a 'short bowel syndrome'. Bile salt depletion may become important. Abnormal motility may also have an effect. Malabsorption in Crohn's disease is often due to a combination of several of these factors.

METABOLISM

Crohn's disease is sometimes referred to as a cause of hypercatabolism. If complicated by severe generalised sepsis or peritonitis, the energy requirements of a patient in bed with Crohn's disease might be expected to amount to as much as 50% more than the basal metabolic rate, but patients with such severe disease are unusual, even in specialised units. Such severe illness occasionally follows a surgical disaster; it will be characterised by a high pyrexia and pulse rate, and the situation will usually be short-lived. As a rule, hypercatabolism seems to be a minor cause of malnutrition in Crohn's disease. We shall return to this later.

LOSSES

Inflammatory bowel disease can result in important losses of protein, water and electrolytes. Such losses will be related to the severity, extent and site of the disease.

Let us consider how these factors interplay in various deficiency syndromes.

ENERGY

It seems likely that, in many patients with Crohn's disease, loss of energy stores is largely due to deficient intake. Malabsorption of carbohydrates, although present in a high proportion of patients with proximal and diffuse small-intestinal disease (Smith, 1969), is seldom so severe as to cause significant reduction in energy supply in the absence of diminished intake. For example, even if a patient on a 100 g fat diet is losing 20 g fat per day as steatorrhoea, 80% is still being absorbed and only 180 kcal are being lost. Absorption of carbohydrate and protein is generally more efficient than that of fat. However, when there has been a massive resection of small bowel, bomb calorimetry of the stools can reveal substantial energy malabsorption. For example, we have recently seen a man in whom about 90 cm of small bowel remain and in whom, on an estimated 3,000 kcal diet, stool energy levels are between 22% and 66% of this value. Energy hypercatabolism is unusual. In our experience at St. Mark's Hospital fairly modest energy inputs of 40–50 kcal/kg body weight/ day result in satisfactory weight gain in nearly all adult patients with Crohn's disease. Le Grix (1976) was able to achieve positive energy balance in patients with inflammatory bowel disease with inputs of 1800–2900 kcal/day. Urea excretion seldom seems higher than would be expected from nitrogen inputs. Figure 9.1 shows urine urea converted to nitrogen output by assuming that 5/6 of urine nitrogen is excreted as urea. It can be seen that inputs above about 8 g nitrogen were usually in excess of urinary nitrogen losses by more than 2 g in patients whose daily total energy input was 2,000 kcal or more.

PROTEIN

Here the situation is less clear. Input is still likely to be important. Nitrogen losses in the faeces of patients with Crohn's disease have not been systematically reported. Clark and Lauder (1969) described patients in whom faecal N amounted to 11 g, 6 g, 9 g and 3 g per 24 hours. In a study of patients with ulcerative colitis, protein losses

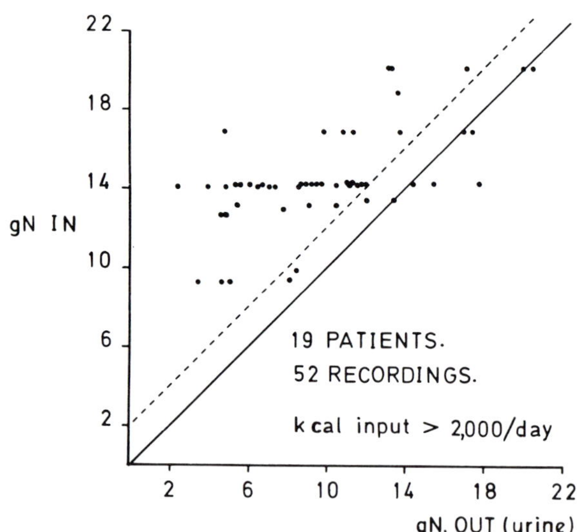

Fig 9.1. *A comparison of nitrogen intake and urinary nitrogen output of patients with Crohn's disease being fed parenterally. The continuous line represents equal N input and urinary N output. Any value above the broken line represents an excess of input over output of more than 2 g N.*

varied with the severity of the disease but could amount to as much as 30 g protein per day (Buckell *et al.*, 1977). It is estimated that a conversion of these results to nitrogen output by a factor of 6·25 would underestimate the stool nitrogen losses by about 1/3 since this proportion of the stool nitrogen is in the form of amino acids or peptides and was not measured by the dye binding technique used. Stool nitrogen will consist not only of dietary nitrogen but, more important in inflammatory bowel disease, also of protein lost from the inflamed mucosa and as desquamated cells. A number of studies have determined the albumin, IgG and ^{59}Fe-iron-dextran clearances from the blood (Steinfeld *et al.*, 1960; Beeken *et al.*, 1972; Jarnum and Jensen, 1975; Jensen and Jarnum, 1976). The fractional 'catabolic' rate of albumin in Crohn's disease varies with the extent of the disease from normal levels (about 10% of the intravascular mass per day) to about 30% per day. This 'catabolic' loss correlates with ^{59}Fe-iron-dextran clearance suggesting that it is, therefore, not truly catabolic but related in part to intestinal loss. These statements seem broadly true of IgG also. The fact that serum levels of IgG are raised while those of albumin are diminished could relate to altered distributions of the proteins between the intravascular and extravascular fluids or to altered rates of synthesis.

Because of the various causes of a low serum albumin in inflammatory bowel disease there is considerable danger in assuming that it correlates with overall protein nutritional status. Anthropometric measurements seem preferable for assessing this.

VITAMINS

While bacterial overgrowth can result in malabsorption of vitamin B_{12}, most B_{12} deficiency in Crohn's disease seems related to the extent of the terminal ileum resected (Dyer *et al.*, 1972) and thus is mostly due to malabsorption. Folate deficiency, however, is more complicated because, although malabsorption may occur, the deficiency may also be seen in disease confined to the colon. Thus, turnover seems important also (Hoffbrand *et al.*, 1968; Dyer *et al.*, 1972).

TRACE ELEMENTS

In Dyer's study, iron deficiency correlated not with disease site but with disease activity (Dyer *et al.*, 1972). It is, therefore, presumably largely due to increased turnover and intestinal losses. The amount of zinc lost from the gastrointestinal tract appears to correlate with the stool weight (Wolman *et al.*, 1979).

Techniques for treating undernutrition

The treatment of undernutrition, or the maintenance of normal nutrition, must be seen as a part of the whole armamentarium for treating the patient. Thus anti-inflammatory drugs may improve absorption and reduce losses or metabolic demands. Steroids may stimulate appetite. Antibiotics may reduce small-intestinal bacterial overgrowth. Resection of diseased bowel may crucially alter the nutritional or metabolic problem, particularly when obstruction is relieved, abscesses are drained, or severely inflamed colon is resected. Priorities, therefore, have to be carefully considered and treatment planned. Specific deficiencies are treated as simply as possible, bearing in mind the cause. Thus, while iron, folic acid and zinc deficiencies can commonly be corrected orally, vitamin B_{12} depletion will need parenteral treatment if the specialised terminal ileum is severely diseased or has been removed. The much rarer deficiencies of fat-soluble vitamins usually require parenteral treatment because they are caused by severe malabsorption following large-scale small-intestinal surgery.

As has already been discussed, we should probably best regard severe hypoalbuminaemia in Crohn's disease as a specific deficiency rather than regarding it primarily as an index of protein malnutrition. Hypoalbuminaemia needs to be corrected if it is so severe that the plasma volume is reduced to such an extent that there is circulatory insufficiency. Treatment is by intravenous infusions of blood, plasma, plasma protein fraction, or albumin. Repeated supply may be necessary if the protein losses from the intestine are not corrected.

In treating P.E.M. or in maintaining normal nutrition, we need to know about ordinary food or to have access to good advice from the dieticians. Weinsier *et al.* (1979) have shown how undernutrition tends to worsen in general medical patients during their stay in hospital. We need to see that hospital food is attractively presented and appropriate for the individual patient's needs. A large number of tests done on patients with Crohn's disease require a period of 'nil by mouth', and ward rounds sometimes have a tendency to coincide with meal-times. It should be remembered, also, that eating becomes psychologically very important to the patient under physical or emotional stress.

When ordinary food alone is not enough, we can supplement it with nutritious drinks or by encouraging the patient to take other easily assimilable foods, such as chocolate or ice-cream, between meals. Of the special products available, we most commonly use Build-up, Complan or Isocal for oral supplements. Is it really beyond the ability of our catering colleagues to make such supplements delicious?

When the oral route is impracticable or insufficient, infusing nutrients into the intestine is next considered. The techniques in use at St. Mark's Hospital have been described elsewhere, together with examples of feeds (Powell-Tuck, 1979). Infusions are given through fine-bore soft silicone rubber tubes (such as the Vygon 6-gauge paediatric tube). The fluids are conveniently dripped or pumped from a re-usable plastic container with an attached giving set (such as the Viomedex bag). They are infused steadily and not in boluses. They can either provide all the nutrient requirements or be used, particularly nocturnally, to supplement the daily intake of ordinary food. The constituents of some of the feeds commonly used in the U.K. are shown in table 9.1. It should be noted that, in many cases, extra sodium, as sodium chloride or bicarbonate, or potassium needs to be added to cover the requirements of the patient with inflammatory bowel disease.

When gastrointestinal feeding is impossible, impracticable or insufficient, intravenous feeding can be used. This has been dealt with in detail in earlier chapters of this book. The techniques and regimens in use at St. Mark's Hospital have been described (Powell-Tuck *et al.*, 1978; Powell-Tuck, 1979) together with a prospective bacteriological study of the methods used (Powell-Tuck *et al.*, 1979). Nutrients (particularly supplemental) can be supplied through peripheral veins for periods of one to two weeks. However, peripheral infusion depends upon the use of large amounts of fat (Intralipid) as energy source since glucose solutions of greater concentration than 5% rapidly cause veins to thrombose. These fat emulsions are expensive and there may be problems of fat utilization in severely ill, particularly septic, patients. The catheters need changing every 24 to 48 hours.

Usually we want to supply all the nutrients a patient needs over periods of several weeks. We then may accept the (approximately 5%) risk of inducing a pneumothorax and insert by blind technique a skin-tunnelled silicone rubber catheter into the superior vena cava or right atrium. If the risk of pneumothorax cannot be taken, the relatively difficult technique of cutting down on the axillary vein or the internal jugular vein, can be used. The fluids are either infused from multiple bottles and bags via a single-piece double giving-set or from a single 3-

Table 9.1. *The major constituents of some commonly used liquid feeds*

Name	Supplier	Quantity	Energy kcal**	Protein (g)	Fat (g)	Na (mmol)	K (mmol)	Ca (mmol)	Mg (mmol)	P (mmol)
Cows milk		1000 ml	650	33	38	22	38	30	5	31
xBuild Up	Carnation Ltd	1 pkt	132	25·6	0·2	5·4	9·8	8·3	0·9	7·9
Complan	Glaxo Ltd		444	20	16	15·2	21·8	18·3	2·9	18·7
*Albumaid	Scientific		305	76	—	54	3·8	7·5	8·5	10·7
*Maxipro	Hospital	100 g	352	88	—	10	11·5	7·5		12·5
*Metabolic Mineral Mix	Supplies Ltd		—	—	—	172	212	205	40	192
*†Triosorbon	BDH Pharmaceutical Ltd	85 g (1 pkt)	400	16·2	16·2	17	17	5·1	3	7·7
Clinifeed 400 Vanilla			400	15	13·4	10·5	12·4	5	2	7·4
Clinifeed 400 Chocolate	Roussel Laboratories Ltd	375 ml (1 tin)	400	15	13·4	10·5	21	5	5·7	9·4
Clinifeed 500 Vanilla			500	30	11·0	12·8	21·6	3·3	1·9	9·0
*Clinifeed LLS			500	22·5	15·0	7·0	12·9	3·4	0·9	6·5
*Ensure	Abbot Laboratories Ltd	235 ml (1 tin)	241	8·7	8·7	7·6	7·7	3·1	2·0	1·6
*†Portagen	Mead Johnson Laboratories	100 g	464	16·5	22·5	9·6	15	11	3·9	10·7
*†Isocal		355 ml (1 tin)	375	12·1	15·7	8·1	12	5·6	3·1	6·1
*†Flexical		100 g	441	9·9	15	6·7	14·1	6·6	3·7	7·1
*Vivonex Standard			300	6·3	0·4	11·2	9	3·3	2·4	1·4
*Vivonex HN	Eaton Laboratories Ltd	80 g 1 pkt	300	12·5	0·3	10·1	5·4	2·0	1·4	0·8

*low lactose †contains MCT xshould be added to milk **kj = kcal × 4·2

litre disposable Viaflex container. Additives to, or mixtures of, fluids are necessary and such preparations are always made by a pharmacist observing strict aseptic technique, working in a 'clean room' under a laminar flow hood.

All the tube feeding and intravenous feeding at St. Mark's Hospital is supervised by a single team, with clinicians, a specialist nursing sister and a dietician working in close liaison with the ward nurses, the pharmacist, the catering department and the biochemical and bacteriological laboratories. We keep detailed daily records of the patient's input of nutrients so that deficiencies and metabolic imbalances such as glucose intolerance or acidosis can be rapidly noted and corrected or prevented. Domiciliary parenteral feeding has already been discussed (Chapter 7). We are increasingly gaining experience with a technique which allows the patient to infuse all the necessary nutrients at home from the disposable 3-litre containers at night, so that he can disconnect the spigot and heparinise the catheter by day and, therefore, continue normal activities unencumbered. This approach can be useful in the very small number of patients with a short bowel following extensive resection for Crohn's disease. Home nocturnal nasogastric feed supplementation can also be considered for the chronically malnourished patient.

Thus our whole approach should be to use the simplest and most effective way of feeding the individual patient, in order to ensure adequate anabolism, to prevent or correct metabolic disturbance and, in the case of intravenous feeding, to prevent or minimise the risk of septicaemia and venous thrombosis. The doctor must realise that it is necessary to organise and coordinate the treatment as well as to prescribe it.

Dietary manipulation as a treatment of Crohn's disease

Table 9.2 shows some of the characteristics of the diet of patients with Crohn's disease before and after the onset of symptoms and compares them with the diet of the general population and control subjects. It can be seen that patients with Crohn's disease eat more refined sugar than normal.

A study of the breakfast habits of patients with Crohn's disease suggested that patients eat more cornflakes, wheat cereals and bran than normal (James, 1977). Three further studies (Rawcliffe and

Table 9.2. *The pre-illness diet of patients with Crohn's disease compared with the diet of subjects in the general population*

	Control subjects		Patients with Crohn's disease		References†
	Number of subjects	*Consumption*	*Number of subjects*	*Pre-illness consumption*	
Energy	*	9·5			1
MJ/day	63	13·4	63	16·4	2
	30	9·6	30	10·4	3
	70	12·3	35	14·4	4
Total	*	273			1
carbohydrate	30	241	30	295	3
g/day	70	261	70	367	4
Total	*	105			1
fat g/day	30	111	30	112	3
	70	137	35	147	4
Total	*	72·3			1
protein	30	74	30	73	3
g/day	70	89	35	96	4
Refined	*	54·5			1
sugar	63	74	63	177	2
g/day	30	65	30	122	3
	70	91	35	156	4
Total	30	19·2	30	17·3	3
fibre g/day	70	22·3	35	26·6	4

*Based on a dietary survey of 7696 households (Reference 1)
† References
  1. National Food Survey (1977)
  2. Martini and Brandes (1976)
  3. Thornton *et al.* (1979)
  4. Kasper and Sommer (1979)

Truelove, 1978; Archer and Harvey, 1978; Mayberry *et al.*, 1978) failed to confirm these findings. The study of Mayberry and co-workers suggested that Crohn's disease sufferers added more sugar to their tea, coffee or cereals than controls.

Heaton and co-workers (1979) treated 32 patients with a diet rich in fibre and unrefined carbohydrate over periods ranging from 18 to 80 months and found that they needed markedly fewer hospital admissions than a retrospectively chosen matched control group (diet treated group 11, controls 34) and spent less time in hospital (111 days) than controls (533 days). These findings could prove to be of great importance, both therapeutically and as a clue to the aetiology of the disease, but they require to be confirmed by prospective studies.

The symptoms of Crohn's disease can include abdominal pain, diarrhoea and a feeling of incomplete evacuation. The addition of fibre to the diet increases faecal bulk. Ispaghula has been shown to improve the symptoms of irritable bowel syndrome (Ritchie and Truelove, 1979) and it seems reasonable to try it or similar preparations for similar symptom patterns attributable to Crohn's disease where active inflammation or obstruction are not marked.

When diarrhoea or salt depletion are attributable to fat malabsorption, reduction of dietary fat to perhaps 60 g/day or less can help by reducing stool volume and sodium content. It has been suggested that, when caloric requirements from fat are necessarily greater than the intake tolerated by the gut, the substitution of triglyceride with fatty acids of 10 carbon atoms or less (medium chain triglyceride M.C.T.) may be beneficial. Such fatty acids are absorbed more readily in the presence of low concentrations of bile salts (as occurs after distal ileal resection) and are transported directly into the portal vein. In practice, although they are occasionally useful, their use as a replacement for dietary fat often does not result in a useful reduction in stool volume and they should be used in individual patients in whom replacement has been demonstrated to cause stool volume or sodium content reduction.

Disaccharide intolerance is common among the general population, and should be borne in mind in patients with persistent diarrhoea. Lactose is by far the most common cause but other disaccharidase deficiencies like sucrase, maltase and trehalase have also been reported. The treatment is to reduce the amount of the relevant disaccharide in the diet.

Bowel rest

It has been hoped that by altering the quality or quantity of the stream of intestinal contents traversing the diseased gut, or by diverting it altogether, healing might be induced. Diversion of the flow by bypass operation passed through a phase of popularity but is now seldom practised because mortality rates following resection have been reduced and there are high re-operation rates following the by-pass procedures (Koudahl *et al.*, 1974; Homan and Dineen, 1978).

In 1965, Truelove and co-workers reported encouraging results with the use of a double-barrelled ileostomy to divert the faeces from a diseased colon. The distal limb of the stoma could be used to instil topical corticosteroids. The experience of St. Mark's Hospital at that time was less encouraging in that of 19 patients treated for colonic or anorectal disease in this way, only two required no further surgery during follow-up and most required resection of the diseased bowel within a year of the diversionary stoma being fashioned (Jones *et al.*, 1966). A further report from the Oxford group included 69 patients (Lee, 1975). The treatment was still regarded as unorthodox, but nevertheless, seemed sometimes beneficial. Unfortunately, there is a high relapse rate when continuity of the intestine is restored. Further opinions have varied (Oberhelman *et al.*, 1968; McIlrath, 1971; Slater *et al.*, 1978) and, at present, in the absence of controlled data, it is not possible to draw further conclusions.

Following an early report by Winitz *et al.* (1970) that a chemically defined (elemental) diet, consisting of amino acids, monosaccharides, electrolytes, trace elements and vitamins, could maintain nutrition over long periods in normal men, with greatly diminished stool output, interest was aroused as to how such a diet might prove useful for sufferers from Crohn's disease. These 'elemental' diets decrease outputs of water, sodium, trypsin and bile acids from the distal ileum (Hill *et al.*, 1975, 1976) but to what extent the effects are due to their liquid presentation, the low fat content, the lack of fibre or the pre-digested state is uncertain. In dogs, elemental diets seem to stimulate pancreatic secretion less than normal food (McArdle *et al.*, 1974) but in humans pancreatic enzyme secretion in response to intrajejunal infusions of liquid feeds appears to correlate with the infusate's nitrogen content and may not depend upon whether or not it is elemental (Vidon *et al.*, 1978). Liquid diets are used principally to maintain or improve nutrition in patients who cannot eat enough normal food because of poor appetite, abdominal pain or partial obstruction. For this purpose, low-osmolar feeds containing oligopeptides rather than high-osmolar elemental feeds containing amino acids may be best (Silk, 1974). Elemental diets can be useful if we wish to reduce colonic faecal output, as, for example, if the perineum is severely diseased. Any advantages claimed for these preparations in healing intestinal fistulae could well be explained by improved nutrition, which can be achieved with simpler, cheaper preparations. Although it is tempting to hypothesize that elemental diets might reduce the inflammation in diseased intestine (perhaps by altering the gut flora or the stimulus, immunological or otherwise, of food), we have no evidence to suggest that this is so. These diets seem at present to be of more use to the research worker than to the clinician.

The presence of food in the gut stimulates secretion of enzymes, fluid, electrolytes, bile and hormones. Motility, blood flow and mucosal cell turnover are increased. Food has a trophic effect on the intestine. We can remove much of this stimulus by stopping the patient eating, and maintaining nutrition parenterally. The place of parenteral feeding in inflammatory bowel disease has already been reviewed elsewhere in this book (Chapter 6). A large number of uncontrolled studies have suggested that 'bowel rest' with parenteral nutrition might be useful in inflammatory bowel disease (Fischer *et al.*, 1973; Anderson and Boyce, 1973; Vogel *et al.*, 1974; Solassol *et al.*, 1974; Greenberg *et al.*, 1976; Galmiche *et al.*, 1977; Rault and Scribner, 1977; Fleming *et al.*, 1977; Driscoll and Rosenberg, 1978; Strobel *et al.*, 1979). One controlled study of bowel rest and parenteral nutrition in 40 patients with acute colitis failed to show a benefit for this treatment (Dickinson *et al.*, 1979). More controlled trials are needed. At present we sometimes stop patients eating a week or two prior to surgery if they are receiving parenteral nutrition for nutritional indications in the belief that we can encourage some degree of resolution of peri-intestinal abscesses, or shrinkage of a dilated obstructed intestine, and thus make the operation simpler for the surgeon. It sometimes seems advisable for the very complicated case to rest the bowel while the patient's nutrition improves over longer periods. I regard the treatment of inflammatory bowel disease by bowel rest as unproven and consider that we should be reluctant to use this form of treatment, with its attendant risks and expense, unless it can be clearly justified on nutritional grounds.

References

Anderson D.L. and Boyce H.W. (1973) *Amer. J. dig. Dis.* **18**, 633.

Archer L.N.J. and Harvey R.F. (1978) *Brit. med. J.* **2**, 540.

Beeken W.L., Busch H.J. and Sylwester D.L. (1972) *Gastroenterology*, **62**, 207–215.

Buckell N.A., Gould S.R., Hernandez M.A., Kohn J., Lennard-Jones J.E., Powell-Tuck J., Riches P.G. and Welch S.G. (1977) *Gut*, **18**, A971.

Clark R.G. and Lauder N.M. (1969) *Brit. J. Surg.* **56**, 736.

Collins J.P., Oxby C.B. and Hill G.L. (1978) *Lancet*, i, 788–791.

Dickinson R.J., Ashton M.G., Axon A.T.R., Goligher J.C., Smith R.C., Yeung C.K. and Hill G.L. (1979) *Gut,* **20**, A445–6.

Driscoll R.H. and Rosenberg I.H. (1978) *Med. Clin. N. Amer.* **62**, 185–201.

Dyer N.H., Child J.A., Mollin D.L. and Dawson A.M. (1972) *Quart. J. Med.* **41**, 419–36.

Fischer J.E., Foster G.S., Abel R.M., Abbott W.M. and Ryan J.A. (1973) *Amer. J. Surg.* **125**, 165–175.

Fleming C.R., McGill D.B. and Berkner S. (1977) *Gastroenterology,* **73**, 1077–1081.

Galmiche J.P., Bihan M. Le., Hecketsweiler P., Colin R., Denis P. and Geffroy Y. (1977) *Med. Chir. Dig.* **6**, 13–17.

Golden M.H.N., Golden B.E., Harland P.S.E.G. and Jackson A.A. (1978) *Lancet,* i, 1226–1228.

Greenberg G.R., Haber G.B. and Jeejeebhoy K.N. (1976) *Gut,* **17**, A828.

Gross R.L., Reid J.V.O., Newberne P.M., Burgess B., Marston R. and Hift W. (1975) *Amer. J. clin. Nutr.* **28**, 225–232.

Halsted J.A., Ronaghy H.A., Abadi P., Haghshenass M., Amirhakemi G.H., Barakat R.M. and Reinhold J.G. (1972) *Amer. J. Med.* **53**, 277–284.

Heaton K.W., Thornton J.R. and Emmett P.M. (1979) *Brit med. J.* **2**, 764–766.

Hill G.L., Mair W.S.J., Edwards J.P., Morgan D.B. and Goligher J.C. (1975) *Gastroenterology,* **68**, 676–682.

Hill G.L., Mair W.S.J., Edwards J.P. and Goligher J.C. (1976) *Brit. J. Surg.* **63**, 133–136.

Hill G.L., Blackett R.L., Pickford I.R. and Bradley J.A. (1977) *Brit. J. Surg.* **64**, 894–896.

Hoffbrand A.V., Stewart J.S., Booth C.C. and Mollin D.L. (1968) *Brit. med. J.* **1**, 71–75.

Homan W.P. and Dineen P. (1978) *Ann. Surg.* **187**, 530–535.

James A.H. (1977) *Brit. med. J.* **1**, 943–5.

Jarnum S. and Jensen K.B. (1975) *Gastroenterology,* **68**, 1433–1444.

Jensen K.B. and Jarnum S. (1976). In *Plasma Protein Turnover,* pp. 45–63, eds. Bianchi R., Mariani G. and McFarlane A.S. Macmillan, London.

Jones J.H., Lennard-Jones J.E. and Lockhart-Mummery H.E. (1966) *Gut,* **7**, 448.

Kasper H. and Sommer H. (1979) *Amer. J. Clin. Nutr.* **32**, 1898–1901.

Kelts D.G., Grand R.J., Shen G., Watkins J.B., Werlin S.L. and Boehme C. (1979) *Gastroenterology,* **76**, 720–727.

Keys A., Brozek J., Aenschel A., Mickelson O. and Taylor H.L. (1950) *The Biology of Human Starvation.* University of Minnesota Press, Minneapolis.

Koudahl G., Kristensen M. and Lenz K. (1974) *Scand. J. Gastroenterol.* **9**, 203–6.

Law D.K., Dudrick S.J. and Abdou N.I. (1973) *Ann. Intern. Med.* **79**, 545–50.

Layden T., Rosenberg J., Nemchausky B., Elson C. and Rosenberg I. (1976) *Gastroenterology,* **70**, 1017–1021.

Leader (1979) *Lancet,* ii, 507–8.

Lee E. (1975) *Ann. Roy. Coll. Surg.* **56**, 94–102.

Le Grix (1976) M.D. Thesis. Faculty of Medicine and Pharmacy, University of Rouen.

Martini G.A. and Brandes J.W. (1976) *Klin. Wochschr.* **54**, 367–371.

Mayberry J.F., Rhodes J. and Newcombe R.G. (1978) *Brit. med. J.* **2**, 1401.

McArdle A.H., Echave W., Brown R.A. and Thompson A.G. (1974) *Amer. J. Surg.* **128**, 690–692.

McIlrath D.C. (1971) *Arch. Surg.* **103**, 308–310.

National Food Survey (1977) *Household food consumption and expenditure. Ministry of Agriculture, Fishery and Foods.* H.M.S.O. London.

Oberhelman H.A., Kohatsu S., Taylor K.B. and Kivel R.M. (1968) *Amer. J. Surg.* **115**, 231–240.

Powell-Tuck J. (1979) *Medicine,* **16**, 825–829.

Powell-Tuck J., Nielsen T., Farwell J.A. and Lennard-Jones J.E. (1978) *Lancet,* **ii**, 825–828.

Powell-Tuck J., Lennard-Jones J.E., Lowes J.A., Twum Danso K. and Shaw E.J. (1979) *J. Clin. Path.* **32**, 549–555.

Rault R.M.J. and Scribner B.J. (1977) *Gastroenterology,* **72**, 1249–1252.

Rawcliffe P.M. and Truelove S.C. (1978) *Brit. med. J.* **2**, 539–40.

Ritchie J.A. and Truelove S.C. (1979) *Brit. med. J.* **1**, 376–378.

Rudman D., Milliken W.J., Richardson T.J., Bixler T.J., Stackhouse W.J. and McGarrity W.C. (1975) *J. clin. Invest.* **55**, 94–104.

Sagar S., Harland P. and Shields R. (1979) *Brit. med. J.* **i**, 293–5.

Silk D.B.A. (1974) *Gut,* **15**, 494–501.

Slater G., Kreel I. and Aufses A.H. (1978) *Ann. Surg.* **188**, 706–709.

Smith A.N. (1969). In *Malabsorption* eds. Girdwood R.H. and Smith A.N. Medical Monographs 4. University Press, Edinburgh.

Solassol C., Joyeux H., Pujol H., Balmes J.L., Cayrol B. and Favier C. (1974) *Arch. Fr. Mal. App. Dig.* **63**, 115–121.

Steiger E., Daly J.M., Allen T.R., Dudrick S.J. and Vars H.M. (1973) *Surgery,* **73**, 686–691.

Steinfeld J.L., Davidson J.D., Gordon R.S. and Greene F.E. (1960) *Amer. J. Med.* **29**, 405–415.

Strobel C.T., Byrne W.J. and Ament M.E. (1979) *Gastroenterology,* **77**, 272–9.

Studley H.O. (1936) *J. Amer. Med. Ass.* **106**, 458.

Thornton J.R., Emmett P.M. and Heaton K.W. (1979) *Brit. med. J.* **2**, 762–4.

Truelove S.C., Ellis H. and Webster C.U. (1965) *Brit. med. J.* **1**, 150.

Vidon N., Hecketsweiler P., Butel J. and Bernier J.J. (1978) *Gut,* **19**, 194–8.

Vogel C.M., Corwin T.R. and Baue A.E. (1974) *Arch. Surg.* **108**, 460–467.

Waterlow J.C., Golden M.H.N. and Picou D. (1977) *Amer. J. clin. Nutr.* **30**, 1333–9.

Waterlow J.C., Golden M.H.N. and Patrick J. (1978). In *Nutrition in the Clinical Management of Disease,* eds. Dickerson J.W.T. and Lee H.A. Edward Arnold. London. pp. 49–71.

Weinsier R.L., Hunker E.M., Krumdieck C.L. and Butterworth C.E. (1979) *Amer. J. Clin. Nutr.* **32**, 418–426.

Winitz M., Seedman D.A. and Graff J. (1970) *Amer. J. Clin. Nutr.* **23**, 525–545.

Wolman S.L., Anderson G.H., Marliss E.B. and Jeejeebhoy K.N. (1979) *Gastroenterology,* **76**, 458–467.

Chapter 10

The case for conservative treatment

M. J. GOODMAN

The forms of treatment available for patients with Crohn's disease comprise the following: resuscitative measures (blood and intravenous fluids) for the shocked or dehydrated patient; a number of specific drugs which suppress or control the disease; other drugs to provide symptomatic relief; dietary measures; psychological and emotional support; and, finally, various surgical procedures. The medical treatment of Crohn's disease can involve any of these forms of treatment other than surgical treatment. It can also take the form of 'masterly inactivity', with the patient being observed, carefully monitored and reassured but with no specific treatment being prescribed.

Specific therapeutic agents

Corticosteroids

The most widely used and most effective drugs for the treatment of active Crohn's disease are the corticosteroids. Hydrocortisone has now been replaced by prednisone and prednisolone (and sometimes methyl-prednisolone) because of their weaker salt-retaining properties. The usual dose of prednisone or prednisolone in treating an attack of Crohn's disease is 15–30 mg daily; the author normally prescribes 20 mg daily in a single morning dose in order to encourage patient compliance and to maintain normal diurnal steroid rhythms (as an evening dose of steroid can interfere with the patient's sleep).

When Crohn's disease affects the rectum and lower sigmoid colon, some benefit can be obtained from the use of local corticosteroid enemas, such as prednisolone retention enemas.

The side effects of the corticosteroids are well known. The patient can develop a Cushingoid facies and habitus; there is protein catabolism with poor healing and thinning of bones and other tissues; there is a tendency to hyperglycaemia; and even with prednisolone and prednisone there remain aldosterone-like effects causing sodium retention, potassium loss and hypertension. Treatment with the corticosteroids suppresses the hypothalamo-pituitary-adrenal axis, preventing the normal physiological secretion of cortisol and, in particular, suppressing the increased cortisol secretion in response to stress.

This suppression can persist for weeks or months following steroid withdrawal; permanent adrenal atrophy with iatrogenic Addison's disease has been known to occur. The corticosteroids are also potent suppressors of growth and their use around the time of puberty can result in irreversible stunting of growth.

Sulphasalazine

Sulphasalazine (salicylazosulphapyridine), which is marketed in the United Kingdom as 'Salazopyrin' and in the United States as 'Azulfidine' and 'SAS-500', consists of 5-aminosalicylic acid linked through a diazo bond to sulphapyridine. This bond is cleaved by colonic bacteria and the active component of the drug in ulcerative colitis has been shown to be the 5-aminosalicylic acid which is released locally in the colon by this cleavage (Azad Khan *et al.*, 1977). The assumption is made that the beneficial action of sulphasalazine in Crohn's disease, which is only seen in Crohn's disease with colonic involvement, occurs in a manner comparable to that in ulcerative colitis.

The optimal dosage of sulphasalazine recommended for maintenance treatment in ulcerative colitis has been shown in careful studies by Azad Khan *et al.* (1980) to be 500 mg four times daily. Lower doses are ineffective and with higher doses there is an increased incidence of side effects (Pounder *et al.*, 1975) without any marked improvement in therapeutic effect. In the absence of detailed studies in Crohn's disease the dosage of sulphasalazine recommended is the same as that in ulcerative colitis, namely, 500 mg four times daily.

The side effects of sulphasalazine include various skin rashes, (including erythema nodosum and photosensitive rashes), nausea (which tends to remit if the patient persists with the drug) and a number of blood dyscrasias. The rarest and most serious of the latter is agranulocytosis which has been reported to be fatal (Thirkettle *et al.*, 1963). More common is haemolytic anaemia, which is usually reversible when the drug is withdrawn. Patients with glucose-6-phosphate dehydrogenase deficiency are particularly prone to developing haemolytic anaemia. With other patients the occurrence of haemolytic anaemia appears to be related to dose (Pounder *et al.*, 1975).

Azathioprine

This drug, which is an immunosuppressant, appears to be only marginally effective in Crohn's disease when used alone. It has been shown in controlled trials to be of value in permitting a more rapid reduction in corticosteroid dosage than would otherwise be the case (Rosenberg *et al.*, 1975). There has also been one study showing a lowering of the relapse rate in patients in remission treated with maintenance azathioprine (O'Donoghue *et al.*, 1978).

The dosage of azathioprine normally recommended in Crohn's disease is 2 mg/kg/day, which means in practice 50 mg two or three times daily. This is well below the dosage used in transplantation and the increased occurrence of certain tumours in transplantation patients treated with azathioprine has not been noted in patients with Crohn's disease (Kinlen *et al.*, 1979). Bone marrow suppression remains the most important side effect of azathioprine and it can be fatal. Pancreatitis is another occasional side effect; it is of interest that sulphasalazine and the corticosteroids are also drugs which can cause pancreatitis. There is a theoretical risk of genetic damage due to azathioprine but there are no definite data on this occurring at the dosage used in Crohn's disease.

The relative value of the corticosteroids, sulphasalazine and azathioprine: Results of the National Cooperative Crohn's Disease Study

A multicentre study of the treatment of Crohn's disease has been taking place in the United States. This, the National Cooperative Crohn's Disease Study (NCCDS), has recently reported its important findings with regard to the relative value of prednisone, sulphasalazine and azathioprine in the treatment of Crohn's disease (Winship *et al.*, 1979; Summers *et al.*, 1979; Singleton *et al.*, 1979a, 1979b; Mekhjian *et al.*, 1979).

By assigning a quantitative Crohn's Disease Activity Index (Best *et al.*, 1976), the NCCDS has shown in a double-blind trial that, for an acute attack of Crohn's disease, prednisone in a dosage of 12–75 mg daily (according to the size of the patient and the severity of the disease) was the most effective of the three drugs studied. Sulphasalazine was the second most effective; and azathioprine was only slightly better than placebo, the differences between these two being less than the conventional level of statistical significance (5%). These were the results of a 4-month course of treatment with a single active drug or placebo. Further analysis of the cases showed that sulphasalazine was ineffective in small-intestinal Crohn's disease but that it was a little better than prednisone in large intestinal Crohn's disease (Summers *et al.*, 1979).

A further trial of prednisone plus sulphasalazine versus prednisone alone actually showed the combined therapy to be slightly inferior to prednisone alone although the differences were not at the 5% level of statistical significance (Singleton *et al.*, 1979b). Results on the use of azathioprine in combination with prednisone or sulphasalazine have not yet been reported by the NCCDS.

Maintenance treatment

The National Cooperative Crohn's Disease Study has also reported on patients in clinical remission treated with prednisone, sulphasalazine, azathioprine or placebo. No significant differences were found, the conclusion being that maintenance drug treatment has no place in Crohn's disease (Summers *et al.*, 1979). This is in contradiction to the findings of O'Donoghue *et al.* (1978) with regard to azathioprine. The NCCDS bears out the findings of Baron *et al.* (1977) that maintenance sulphasalazine does not prevent relapse, in contradistinction to the prophylactic value of maintenance sulphasalazine in ulcerative colitis (Dissanayake and Truelove, 1973).

Other therapeutic agents

Metronidazole (Flagyl), an antimicrobial agent specific for colonic Bacteroides, has been reported to be beneficial in occasional cases of Crohn's disease (Ursing and Kamme, 1975). It has recently been reported as being of value in the healing of perianal Crohn's disease (Bernstein *et al.*, 1980). In a double-blind controlled trial of 20 cases in Sweden, metronidazole was no better than a placebo (Blichfeldt *et al.*, 1976).

Disodium Cromoglycate is marketed in the United Kingdom in an oral form (Nalcrom) for the treatment of ulcerative colitis. It was shown by Grundman *et al.* (1978) to be of no value in Crohn's disease.

6-Mercaptopurine has been used by Present *et al.* (1980) with apparently good results. When azathioprine is given, it is converted into 6-mercapto-purine, so it is to be expected that these two drugs will give similar results.

Cyclophosphamide was shown to be of no benefit in Crohn's disease in a trial by Brooke *et al.* (1970).

Levamisole, a stimulant of immune responses, was tried by Segal *et al.* (1977) in eight patients with Crohn's disease in a double-blind cross-over trial. Although the authors claimed 'excellent benefit', two of their patients developed a severe arthritis which remitted when the drug was withdrawn.

BCG immune stimulation has been tried as a treatment for Crohn's disease but was shown to be of no value in a trial by Burnham *et al.* (1979).

Transfer Factor has been investigated as therapy for Crohn's disease by Vicary and others. As a result of a formal trial, Vicary *et al.* (1979) have now concluded that transfer factor confers no benefit in Crohn's disease.

Symptomatic treatment

This should always be considered an essential part of the medical treatment of Crohn's disease, which cannot be deemed to have failed without an attempt at symptomatic therapy if pain or bowel distur-bance are the patient's principal problems. Conventional analgesics are often required, although, in the presence of extensive active Crohn's colitis, the opiates should be avoided because of their tendency, as in ulcerative colitis, to cause toxic dilatation of the colon. Also, the constipating tendencies of the opiates, including pentazocine (Fortral), codeine and dihydrocodeine (DF-118), should be remembered before these drugs are prescribed to a patient with an incipient colonic or small bowel obstruction.

Not only do codeine, loperamide ('Imodium') and diphenoxylate ('Lomotil') relieve diarrhoea as a symptom but they have now been shown to stimulate a measurable degree of additional salt and water retention in the small intestine (Binder, 1976). These drugs are also liable to precipitate toxic dilatation in ulcerative colitis and, by analogy, should probably be avoided in patients with severely active Crohn's disease of the colon.

Bowel rest, parenteral alimentation and elemental diets

The intensive intravenous regimen of Truelove and Jewell (1974) for ulcerative colitis has been used by these physicians and others in the treatment of severe Crohn's disease, particularly Crohn's disease of the colon. This regimen comprises bowel rest with intravenous hydration and alimentation, intravenous corticosteroids in high dosage and (a debated component) an intravenous broad-spectrum antibiotic. Many physicians omit the antibiotic, without apparent detriment, and it was thought by some that bowel rest in Truelove and Jewell's regimen might be as important as the intravenous steroids. Jeejeebhoy and others have attempted to rest the bowel for prolonged periods of up to several months with the use of parenteral alimentation (Greenberg *et al.*, 1976). Notable remissions have occurred but concern about atrophy of the villi of the rested bowel has led to the use of elemental diets of monosaccharides, amino acids and oligopeptides with equally favourable results (Goode *et al.*, 1976). However, it is by no means certain that the elemental diet confers benefit by virtue of resting the bowel. The opportunity to restore nutrition in a depleted patient by means of an elemental diet, or by parenteral alimentation, is the probable reason for the benefit of these forms of therapy; the lack of faecal residue with these diets will relieve the patient of faecal diarrhoea and presumably thereby permit the tolerance of more calories and amino acids than with normal foods.

Treatment with the elemental preparation Vivonex has been demonstrated to cause a 50 per cent decrease in the loss of protein in the faeces (Logan *et al.*, 1979). Whilst restoration of optimal nutrition is without doubt beneficial, there is little evidence to support hyper-alimentation in Crohn's disease, with the patient receiving an abundance of nutritional components beyond the quantities required to restore the disease-induced losses (Greenberg *et al.*, 1976).

Dietary measures

American gastroenterologists from Bargen to Kirsner have recommended low-residue diets for patients with ulcerative colitis and Crohn's disease, although without experimental supportive evidence. When a patient with Crohn's disease has a very narrow segment, particularly in the small intestine, high-roughage foods may possibly obstruct at such a point and it would appear logical to advise the patient to avoid seeds, skins and stringy foods, such as celery and perhaps lettuce. The author has had patients who can recall having eaten high-roughage foods shortly before developing obstructive symptoms but one cannot be certain that this is cause and effect. The traditional prescription of a low-residue diet in Crohn's disease has now been questioned by Heaton *et al.* (1979) who have reported improvement in the clinical condition of Crohn's disease patients treated with a *high*-residue diet. Further studies are clearly required but this opens the possibility of a *volte face* in the dietary recommendations in Crohn's disease. For the time being, it may be best to advise patients to eat what they fancy, and a lot of what they fancy if they are nutritionally depleted; if they do have a narrow segment of bowel, they should continue to avoid foods which are liable to cause obstruction.

Treatment of complications

Certain of the complications of Crohn's disease require specific therapy *per se.* Of the local complications, *fistulae* have been treated successfully by Brooke *et al.* (1970) with azathioprine and by Rault and Scribner (1977) and others with elemental diets and parenteral alimentation, but these have not been controlled observations.

Of the peripheral manifestations of colonic Crohn's disease (which are identical to those of ulcerative colitis), the various forms of *arthritis* may require specific therapy with salicylates, other nonsteroidal anti-inflammatory agents or even corticosteroids. *Ankylosing spondylitis* is sometimes helped by treatment with phenylbutazone. The author has experience of fissured ulcers in patients with Crohn's disease bleeding heavily following the use of indomethacin for arthritic complications and so this drug should probably be avoided. *Uveitis* and *conjunctivitis* may require the use of ocular steroids and other agents. The presence of *chronic active hepatitis* in association with Crohn's disease may be the reason for giving the patients corticosteroids with or without azathioprine.

Surgical treatment

Besides local perianal procedures, the drainage of abscesses and the performance of diagnostic laparotomy in a doubtful case (the latter most often in a patient presenting with acute terminal ileitis), the surgical treatment of Crohn's disease consists of the attempted removal of as much of the disease as possible. This may be impracticable if the disease is very extensive in the small intestine; the patient must be left with the maximum possible length of functioning small bowel. In the case of gastric and duodenal Crohn's disease, resection is less often feasible than with the much more common Crohn's disease of the small and large intestine.

When the disease involves the rectum, the resection of all involved areas will necessarily leave the patient with an ileostomy or a colostomy. If the rectum is uninvolved, or only mildly affected, an end-to-end anastomosis in one or two stages may be performed, leaving the patient with a functioning anus. Ileorectal anastomosis for Crohn's disease of the colon can be a satisfactory procedure even in extensive colonic Crohn's disease provided the rectum is relatively spared (Weterman and Peña, 1976).

Indications for surgery

The indications for surgical resection in Crohn's disease can be divided into absolute indications and considered decisions.

The absolute indications for surgery are:—

Complete and irreversible intestinal obstruction;
Perforation leading to peritonitis;

Uncontrollable haemorrhage;
Abscess formation (drainage rather than resection may be adequate);
Carcinoma complicating Crohn's disease.
The relative indications for resective surgery are:—
Incomplete or recurrent intestinal obstruction;
Fistula formation;
Ureteric obstruction (Present *et al.*, 1969), although the indications for this may not be as rigorous as once thought (Siminovitch and Fazio, 1980);
In the treatment of some of the complications of Crohn's disease of the colon, such as chronic liver disease, which possibly improves following total colectomy (Eade *et al.*, 1970);
Failure of medical therapy.
Where the indications are only relative, the general condition of the patient and the anatomical extent and the severity of the disease all naturally affect the decision regarding surgery. The indication of failed medical therapy is clearly a matter of opinion in an individual case and the criteria to define failure of medical therapy will depend on whether the prevailing view is conservative or aggressive with regard to surgery in Crohn's disease.

Considerations regarding surgery

In favour of proceeding to surgery even when further medical therapy is a practicable alternative are the following arguments:
The diseased part of the bowel is removed.
The dangers of the drugs used in medical therapy are avoided.
There may be some relief of peripheral complications.
The arguments against performing surgery in a doubtful case can be summarised as follows:
Mortality and morbidity can result from surgery.
Functioning absorbing small intestine is irretrievably removed.
In many cases a temporary or a permanent ileostomy or colostomy is required.
The disease is not ablated and there is an ever present risk of recurrence. Some hold the view, unsubstantiated as yet by any published evidence, that the disease can recur in a segment of intestine into which the disease would not have spread if surgery had been avoided.

Postoperative recurrence

Following apparent surgical extirpation of the disease, there is an increasing tendency with time for Crohn's disease to recur. Even six weeks following resection, recurrences are known to occur. Greenstein *et al.* (1975) reported on the recurrence rate in patients operated on at the Mount Sinai Hospital, New York. 15 years after resection, there was evidence of clinical recurrence in 95% of cases and 90% of the patients had required a further operation. The experience of other centres is in accordance with that of Mount Sinai although recurrence rates vary down to rates about 30% less than those experienced by Greenstein *et al.* On the whole, 50% of patients will have relapsed after about 5 years.

In the National Cooperative Crohn's Disease Study the recurrence rate was noticeably less for Crohn's disease confined to the colon than for small intestinal and ileocaecal Crohn's disease (Mekhjian *et al.*, 1979). Fawaz *et al.* (1976) consider that Crohn's disease of the colon has quite a low recurrence rate following panproctocolectomy but the tendency to recurrence of Crohn's disease involving the small intestine is not doubted.

Krause *et al.* (1971) claimed that the recurrence rate was lowered if a wider resection was performed but their evidence was retrospective and they did not compare cases of similar severity. Papaioannou *et al.* (1979) now provide evidence that the length of normal bowel removed adjacent to the diseased area does not affect the recurrence rate and hence argue for removing the minimum amount of uninflamed intestine.

Crohn's disease as a diffuse disease

The pronounced tendency of Crohn's disease to recur following resection of that part of the bowel with obvious disease suggests that the disease is more diffuse than is apparent.

Korelitz and Sommers (1977) reported that careful examination of rectal biopsy specimens from patients with Crohn's disease who apparently had rectal sparing as judged sigmoidoscopically would often reveal histological abnormalities. Goodman *et al.* (1976) found abnormal features even in those rectal biopsies that had been reported as histologically normal by expert pathologists. They measured glucosamine synthetase levels in these apparently normal biopsies and found elevation of the levels of this enzyme. Quantitative histological measurements on these biopsies revealed a fourfold increase in the plasma cell density in the lamina propria and also an increase in the size of the lamina propria itself. Dunne *et al.* (1977) showed reduced levels of disaccharidases in histologically normal small bowel biopsies from patients with Crohn's disease elsewhere in the bowel.

The conclusion drawn from these studies is that Crohn's disease is a diffuse disease of the small and large intestine (and perhaps of the oral, oesophageal and gastric mucosa also) which manifests itself from time to time with macroscopic lesions of varying extent. Surgical removal of these macroscopic lesions would not be expected to remove the disease.

Medical therapy or surgical therapy: Results of the University of Chicago Study

The study

There have been no controlled trials of medical versus surgical therapy in patients with Crohn's disease in whom the indications for surgery have not been strong. Goodman and Kirsner (1979) have studied retrospectively all patients attending the Gastroenterology Clinics of the University of Chicago for the first time with Crohn's disease in the five year period 1970–1974, excluding patients who had had a previous bowel resection and excluding those in whom there was macroscopic rectal involvement on sigmoidoscopy, or particularly extensive small bowel disease, or gastroduodenal disease. In other words, the only patients considered were those in whom a resection with an anastomosis would have been feasible. The study was confined to those patients in whom a decision for surgery was not made within one month of first attendance and it was restricted to patients followed up at the University of Chicago for at least six months.

The results of this study may be of relevance to the question of when to operate on patients with Crohn's disease. It represents the experience of a well known group of gastroenterologists with a renowned leaning to medical therapy rather than surgical therapy. Dr Kirsner and his associates have always been reluctant to recommend surgery for their patients with inflammatory disease.

Method of analysis

From analysis of the hospital case notes each patient was given a clinical grade of A (well), B (fair) or C (unwell) for their first visit and for their subsequent six-monthly visits (taking the clinic visit or hospital admission date nearest to each half-year from the initial visit). Grade C was assigned if the patient came under this grade by virtue of any one of the clinical and laboratory criteria that were under consideration in this study (Table 10.1). Similarly, grade B was assigned if the patient qualified for that grade by any one of the criteria for that grade but was not in grade C; patients assigned grade A were well by all the criteria.

Patients requiring surgery

Out of 83 patients in the study, who were followed up for a mean period of 3·2 years, surgical resection was recommended for 30 patients and the remaining 53 patients were managed medically, apart from

Table 10.1. *University of Chicago Crohn's Disease Study. Criteria used for clinical grading at each six-monthly clinic visit*

Grade	A (Well)	B (Fair)	C (Unwell)
General condition	Well, or unwell from unrelated disease	Fair	Not well
Stools per 24 hr	3 or less	4 or 5	6 or more
Abdominal pain	Occasional & mild	Often but mild	More than mild
Arthritis or backache	None, or due to unrelated disease	Mild	Significant
Malaise	None	Occasional	Persistent
Rectal bleeding	None	Occasional	Frequent
Nausea, vomiting	None	None	Present
Perianal fistula	Tiny	Present	Severe
Other fistula	None	Not draining	Draining
Haemoglobin	More than 11·0 gm	8·5−11·0 gm	Less than 8·5 gm
SGOT	<25% above normal	25% above normal	
Hospitalization in previous 4 months	None, or due to unrelated disease	None, or due to unrelated disease	For Crohn's disease
Medicines in previous 4 months	<10 mg prednisone daily; No azathioprine	10 mg prednisone daily or more; Azathioprine	

perianal operations in a few cases. One of the 30 patients in whom surgery was recommended refused to have the operation and changed doctor. When telephoned five years later this patient was found to be in good health and had not had the operation. Four out of the 29 patients on whom a resection was performed required a second resection during the follow-up period. The indications for the 33 resections that were performed are listed in Table 10.2. It can be seen that failure of medical therapy was the indication for eight of these resections. Failure of medical therapy could be retrospectively defined as failure to respond to three weeks of in-patient medical treatment in the six months preceding a decision to recommend surgery, including one week's treatment in the month preceding surgery. The patient who refused surgery had been recommended to have the operation for failure of medical therapy and in his case these stated criteria for failed medical therapy had not been satisfied. This patient could be described as the exception that proved the rule.

Results

Clearly, the 30 patients in whom surgery was recommended could not be considered strictly comparable to the 53 patients treated medically. Of the latter group (designated the medical group), patients in grades A or B on their first visit generally remained in these grades through-

Table 10.2. *University of Chicago Crohn's Disease Study. Indications for surgery in the 33 bowel resections carried out at or on the recommendation of the University of Chicago*

	No. of Operations
Intestinal obstruction — acute, subacute or recurrent	13
Perforation	2
Fistulae — enterocutaneous	1
enterovaginal	1
enteroenteric	4
Ureteric obstruction	4
Failure of medical therapy	8
Total	33

out follow-up (Table 10.3). Patients who start out with mild disease are seen to continue to do relatively well, as has been shown for ulcerative colitis (Edwards and Truelove, 1963).

When patients who were in Grade C at their first visit are compared according to whether they are in the medical group or the surgical group (the latter term referring to the 30 patients for whom surgery was recommended), it can be seen, first of all, that the medically treated patients distribute themselves fairly evenly between the three clinical grades at their subsequent visits, this being the case even more than four years after their first attendance (Table 10.4). For the surgical group patients their preoperative and postoperative grades are shown separately in Table 10.4. Not surprisingly, the patients were doing badly preoperatively; this is why they were selected for operation. When their postoperative visits are considered, it can be seen that they then distribute themselves between the three clinical grades in a manner similar to the distribution of the medically treated patients. The only death in the series occurred in the surgical group.

The principal result of this study is that the surgically treated patients did no better after their operation than did the patients of similar clinical severity at their initial presentation in whom resective surgery was avoided. For the surgically treated patients the operation improved their clinical status after it had become particularly severe. It did not make the patients any better, on the whole, than the medically treated group of patients.

The experience at Birmingham General Hospital

In the University of Chicago study two thirds of patients were classed as well or fairly well at their six-monthly follow-up visits. This can be compared with the experience at Birmingham General Hospital reported by Higgens and Allen (1979). Out of 238 patients with Crohn's disease followed up for a mean period of 16·6 years, 210 underwent a surgical resection. At their latest attendance, 161 of these patients were well and symptom-free and a further 20 were taking corticosteroids. Seventeen had died from Crohn's disease and there were 17 apparently unrelated deaths. The older mean age of onset of Crohn's disease in the Birmingham patients (31 years) compared to the Chicago patients (21 years) might be expected to imply that the Chicago patients would have a worse prognosis if a young age of onset has the same bad effect

Table 10.3. *University of Chicago Crohn's Disease Study. Numbers of patient-visits (6 monthly visits) in each clinical grade for the non-surgical patients who were graded A or B on their first visits*

Clinical grade	Follow-up period			
	6 & 12 months	*18 & 24 months*	*30, 36, 42 & 48 months*	*54–84 months*
A (Well)	5	10	8	5
B (Fair)	17	7	7	5
C (Unwell)	2	2	3	1

on prognosis as has been found in ulcerative colitis (Edwards and Truelove, 1963). The broad similarity in prognosis between the Chicago and Birmingham patients does not appear to resolve the question as to whether more surgery or less surgery is desirable in Crohn's disease but it appears simply to vindicate careful treatment by experienced and dedicated physicians and surgeons.

Table 10.4. *University of Chicago Crohn's Disease Study. Numbers of patient-visits (6 monthly visits) in each clinical grade for patients graded C on their first visit (A = well, B = fair, C = unwell)*

	Clinical grade	Follow-up period			
		6 & 12 months	*18 & 24 months*	*30, 36, 42 & 48 months*	*54–84 months*
Nonsurgical	A	11	13	20	13
group	B	39	24	26	13
	C	20	16	21	11
Surgical	A	1	0	0	0
group: preop.	B	14	3	2	0
visits	C	21	10	6	4
Surgical	A	0	8	13	7
group: postop.	B	1	7	14	8
visits	C	1	3	9	8

Conclusion

In this Chapter there has been no clear answer to the question as to whether a patient presenting with ileocaecal Crohn's disease should be managed initially medically or surgically. This, the 64 000 dollar question in Crohn's disease, will require a large prospective controlled trial. For the moment it seems that medical and surgical therapy may be of comparable efficacy in the case of the patient in whom resection with anastomosis is feasible and in whom there is no absolute or overwhelming indication for surgery. In these circumstances, it seems that the patient should not be subjected to an avoidable ablative operation and that medical therapy should be preferred if the indications for medical and surgical treatment appear equal.

References

Azad Khan A.K., Howes D.T., Piris J. and Truelove S.C. (1980) *Gut,* **21** (in press).

Azad Khan A.K., Piris J. and Truelove S.C. (1977) *Lancet,* **ii**, 892.

Baron J.H., Bennett P.N., Lennard-Jones J.E., Swarbrick E.T., Coghill N.F., Stewart J.S., Dowling R.H., Neale G., Avery Jones F., Misiewicz J.J., Langman M.J., Milton-Thompson G. and Watkinson G. (1977) *Gut,* **18**, 69.

Bernstein L.H., Frank M.S., Brandt L.J. and Boley S.J. (1980) *Gastroenterology,* **79**, 357.

Best W.R., Becktel J.M., Singleton J.W. and Kern F. (1976) *Gastroenterology,* **70**, 439.

Binder H.J. (1976) *Gastroenterology,* **70**, 864.

Blichfeldt J.P., Blomhoff J.P., Myhre E. and Gjone E. (1976) *Scand. J. Gastroenterol. Suppl.* **38**, 100.

Brooke B.N., Javett S.L. and Davison O.W. (1970) *Lancet,* **ii**, 1050.

Burnham W.R., Lennard-Jones J.E., Hecketsweiler P., Colin R. and Geffroy Y. (1979) *Gut,* **20**, 229.

Dissanayake A.S. and Truelove S.C. (1973) *Gut,* **14**, 923.

Dunne W.T., Cooke W.T. and Allen R.N. (1977) *Gut,* **18**, 290.

Eade M.N., Cooke W.T. and Brooke B.N. (1970) *Ann. intern. Med.* **72**, 489.

Edwards F.C. and Truelove S.C. (1963) *Gut,* **4**, 299.

Fawaz K.A., Glotzer D.J., Goldman H., Dickersin G.R., Gross W. and Patterson J.F. (1976) *Gastroenterology,* **71**, 372.

Goode A., Hawkins T., Fegetter J.G.W. and Johnstone I.D.A. (1976) *Lancet,* **i**, 122.

Goodman M.J. and Kirsner J.B. (1979) *Gastroenterology,* **76**, 1140.

Goodman M.J., Skinner J.M. and Truelove S.C. (1976) *Lancet,* **i**, 275.

Greenberg G.R., Haber G.B. and Jeejeebhoy K.N. (1976) *Gut,* **17**, 828.

Greenstein A.J., Sachar D.B., Pasternack B.S. and Janowitz H.D. (1975) *New Engl. J. Med.* **293**, 685.

Grundman M.J., Williams S.E. and Turnberg L.A. (1978) *Gut,* **19**, 963.

Heaton K.W., Thornton J.R. and Emmett P. (1979) *Brit. med. J.* **2**, 764.

Higgens C. and Allen R.N. (1979) *Gut,* **20**, A940.

Kinlen L.J., Sheil A.G.R., Peto J. and Doll R. (1979) *Brit. med. J.* **2**, 1461.

Korelitz B.I. and Sommers S.C. (1977) *J. Amer. med. Ass.* **237**, 2742.

Krause U., Bergman L. and Norlen B.J. (1971) *Scand. J. Gastroenterol.* **6**, 97.

Logan R.F.A., Gillon J., Ferrington C. and Ferguson A. (1979) *Gut,* **20**, A905.

Mekhjian H.S., Switz D.M., Watts H.D., Deren J.J., Katon R.M. and Beman F.M. (1979) *Gastroenterology,* **77**, 907.

O'Donoghue D.P., Dawson A.M., Powell-Tuck J., Bown R.L. and Lennard-Jones J.E. (1978) *Lancet,* **i**, 955.

Papaioannou N., Piris J., Lee E.C.G. and Kettlewell M.G.W. (1979) *Gut,* **20**, A916.

Pounder R.E., Craven E.R., Henthorn J.S. and Ballantyne J.M. (1975) *Gut,* **16**, 181.

Present D.H., Korelitz B.I., Wisch N., Glass, J.L., Sachar D.B. and Pasternack B.S. (1980) *New Engl. J. Med.* **302**, 981.

Present D.H., Rabinowitz J.G., Banks P.A. and Janowitz H.D. (1969) *New Engl. J. Med.* **280**, 523.

Rault R.M.J. and Scribner B.H. (1977) *Gastroenterology,* **72**, 1249.

Rosenberg J.L., Levin B., Wall A.J. and Kirsner J.B. (1975) *Amer. J. dig. Dis.* **20**, 721.

Segal A.W., Levi A.J. and Loewi G. (1977) *Lancet,* **ii**, 382.

Siminovitch J.M.P. and Fazio V.W. (1980) *Amer. J. Surg.* **139**, 95.

Singleton J.W., Law D.H., Kelley M.L., Mekhjian H.S. and Sturdevant R.A.L. (1979a) *Gastroenterology,* **77**, 870.

Singleton J.W., Summers R.W., Kern F., Becktel J.M., Best W.R., Hansen R.N. and Winship D.H. (1979b) *Gastroenterology,* **77**, 897.

Summers R.W., Switz D.M., Sessions J.T., Becktel J.M., Best W.R., Kern F. and Singleton J.W. (1979) *Gastroenterology,* **77**, 847.

Thirkettle J.L., Gough K.R. and Read A.E. (1963) *Lancet,* **i**, 1395.

Truelove S.C. and Jewell D.P. (1974) *Lancet,* **i**, 1067.

Ursing B. and Kamme C. (1975) *Lancet,* **i**, 775.

Vicary F.R., Chambers J.D. and Dhillon P. (1979) *Gut,* **20**, 408.

Weterman I.T. and Peña A.S. (1976) *Scand. J. Gastroenterol.* **11**, 185.

Winship D.H., Summers R.W., Singleton J.W., Best W.R., Becktel J.M., Lenk J.F. and Kern F. (1979) *Gastroenterology,* **77**, 827.

Chapter 11
Surgical treatment

J. C. GOLIGHER

Crohn's disease can occur anywhere in the alimentary tract from the mouth to the anus. Exceptionally, it may occur quite remote from the alimentary system, although usually in association with a concomitant gastro-intestinal lesion. Nevertheless, it is essentially an *intestinal* complaint (Goligher, 1980). However, even within the bowel its distribution and appearances can differ enormously from case to case, with single or multiple lesions of varying location and extent. Any clinico-pathological classification of such an ailment is thus bound to be somewhat arbitrary, but it is perhaps helpful in considering the results of treatment to distinguish between two main forms of the disease:—

One is so-called *classical Crohn's disease,* as described by Crohn, Ginzburg and Oppenheimer in 1932, which affects chiefly the small intestine, usually the lower ileum, with or without some extension into the caecum or right colon.

The other form is *Crohn's disease mainly or entirely of the large bowel,* in the recognition and definition of which we owe so much to the writings of Lockhart-Mummery and Morson (1960, 1964). In this variety, the disease may be confined absolutely to the colon and rectum or may extend a variable distance in continuity or in 'skip' lesions to the small bowel, but the main emphasis is on the large intestine. Again, the distribution may range from relatively localized segments of disease to, more usually, extensive involvement, which may at first sight resemble macroscopically ordinary ulcerative colitis. One pattern of involvement that occurs in about 25—30% of the patients with large bowel Crohn's disease warrants special mention because of its bearing on the choice of surgical treatment. In it there is heavy implication of the ascending and transverse colon and some involvement of the lower ileum, but the left side of the colon is less

                         J. C. Goligher

severely affected and, as the disease is traced distally, it gradually
peters out in the lower descending or upper sigmoid colon, leaving
what appears grossly and sigmoidoscopically to be a normal rectum and
distal sigmoid.

My own personal experience of Crohn's disease, which now comprises just under 600 patients, was last critically surveyed in 1977—78
when I had treated 517 intestinal cases, classified according to their
initial manifestations into 165 of mainly small bowel type and 352 of
mainly large bowel type (Table 11.1) (Goligher, 1979; 1980). This
dominance by the large bowel variety presumably springs at least in
part from my long-standing interest in ulcerative colitis and colorectal
surgery in general, which leads to many patients being referred to me
with what was presumed by the family practitioner or consultant
physician to be ordinary colitis but was really Crohn's colitis. I do not
imagine that the figures shown here are representative of the relative
distribution of small and large bowel Crohn's disease in the average
general surgical practice. They are more comparable with those obtaining at St. Mark's Hospital, though within the large bowel group there
are, I know, fewer with disease confined strictly to the anal region and
rectum — the so-called *anorectal Crohn's disease* — than at St. Mark's,
the proportion with very distal large bowel disease in my series of
large bowel cases being 12·8% as against roughly 25% at St. Mark's
Hospital (Ritchie and Lennard-Jones, 1976).

Crohn's disease mainly of the small bowel

Of 165 patients suffering from mainly small bowel disease, 133 or 81%

Table 11.1. *Distribution of lesions in 517 cases of intestinal Crohn's Disease in the author's practice, 1960—78*

Distribution of Lesions		
In small bowel alone	102	
		165
In small and large bowel — mainly s. bowel	63	
In small and large bowel — mainly l. bowel	131	
		352
In large bowel alone	221	

came to surgical treatment. Many of these cases had been referred initially for operation after periods of medical management elsewhere and a few had conservative treatment for a time under my care before they were finally brought to operation. Also, it should be pointed out that a number of them had already undergone one or more operations in other centres and that some who underwent primary or subsequent surgical treatment eventually came to yet further operations. That is why 146 operations – primary and subsequent – were employed in the treatment of 133 patients (Table 11.2).

Choice of operation

As can be seen, the keynote to the operative measures used was excision. Sometimes this was of small bowel alone (usually in the form of a terminal ile-ectomy), or, far more commonly, this manoeuvre combined with a limited right hemi-colectomy. Rarely, more elaborate and extensive operations were necessary. It will be noted that the once popular procedure of bypass with unilateral exclusion by means of an end-to-side ileo-transverse colostomy, much practised at one stage by

Table 11.2. *Operations used in the treatment of 98 cases with primary and 48 cases with recurrent Crohn's Disease of small bowel, 1960–78 (from Goligher, 1980)*

Operation employed	Primary	Repeat
Small bowel resection (SBR)	5	3
SBR + right colectomy (RC)	75	34
SBR + RC + ileostomy	3	5
SBR + RC + separation or resection of sigmoid	6	0
SBR + subtotal colectomy + ileorectal anastomosis	0	1
SBR + complete protocolectomy + ileostomy	0	1
Small bowel bypass	5	1
Other operations	4	3
All operations	98	48
Operative deaths	4 (4·1%)	4 (8·3%)

the surgeons of the Mount Sinai Hospital, New York City (Garlock *et al.*, 1951), was hardly used at all. This was not because of any certain knowledge that it is less effective than resection, but simply because of the swing of surgical fashion towards resection in the last 20 years or so. In fact there are no good comparative data on the relative merits of these two types of operation. In most large published series of cases treated surgically for small bowel Crohn's disease, there are at least a few patients who were submitted to bypass with exclusion. Usually they have not done quite so well as those treated by resection, but these are not fair comparisons, for often the patients selected for bypass had very extensive lesions with much involvement of the mesenteric nodes, producing a thick oedematous mesentery and making them unsuitable for resection. The odds have thus been rather heavily loaded against bypass in comparisons of it with resection. (Atwell *et al.*, 1965; Goligher *et al.*, 1971; Williams, 1971; Koudahl *et al.*, 1974; Young *et al.*, 1975). My own guess is that, in a properly controlled trial, bypass with exclusion would be found to be less effective than resection, but that remains to be established. It would also appear from a recent report by Greenstein *et al.* (1978) at the Mount Sinai Hospital that a further drawback to the bypass procedure is the development after many years of carcinoma in the excluded segment of diseased bowel.

Operative mortality

The operative mortality is in accord with what has been published in several other series (van Patter *et al.*, 1954, 3·9%; Barbour *et al.*, 1962, 2·4%; Williams, 1971, 3·9%; and Krause *et al.*, 1971, 5·6%), it being not unnaturally somewhat higher after repeat interventions than after primary operations. Hopefully, the mortality would be rather lower at the present day because of the better nutritional support and more effective antibiotics now available.

Recurrence

The analysis of recurrence will be confined to those patients who were treated by resection and had their primary operation under my care. It is clear that the incidence of recurrent disease increases the longer the period of follow-up, for the recurrence rate in 81 cases followed for 1– 18 years was 22%, that for 48 patients followed at least 5 years 30%, that for 26 patients having 10 or more years of follow-up 47% and that for 14 patients achieving a 5–18 year follow-up 64% — a progression that has been noted by many previous authors (van Petter *et al.*, 1954; Barbour *et al.*, 1962; Bergman and Krause, 1977).

Again, as observed by many others, the site of the majority of the recurrences in this series was just proximal to the anastomosis. This finding has prompted the thought that the incidence of recurrence might conceivably be reduced by a more radical type of initial resection, as advocated notably by Wenckert (1971) and Krause (1979, personal communication), with excision of at least 20–30 cm of apparently normal bowel proximal and distal to the obvious diseased portion, plus a wide deep V-shaped excision of mesentery. Unfortunately there have been no properly controlled trials on this issue, with random allocation of patients either to a very limited removal or to a more radical resection. But Bergman and Krause (1977) have produced some information relevant to this theme from 2 different hospitals in the region of Uppsala, in one of which the surgical policy has been to do a very limited excision whilst in the other a much more radical type of operation of the Wenckert (1971) type has been routinely favored. A 7–19 year follow-up revealed an 84% recurrence rate after the more restricted operation as against just under 30% after the wider excision. But whether these data provide a valid comparison of the efficacy of the two types of procedure is uncertain. Probably most British surgeons adopt a compromise between these two extremes in carrying out a resection for Crohn's enteritis, as I do myself. That is to say, the lesion is resected with proximally and distally a 7–10 cm margin of normal bowel as judged from the serosal surface. Then, before proceeding to the anastomosis, the excised portion of bowel is immediately opened up and its interior examined macroscopically to make sure that the disease is not more extensive on the mucosal than the serosal aspect. If necessary, more bowel is resected to get well clear of the disease and any further segment excised is also immediately examined in the same way. I have not usually had frozen section histological study of the ends of the resection specimen, but have relied on naked-eye examination. As for enlarged mesenteric nodes, I have usually removed these as widely as can be accomplished by a deep excision of mesentery not necessitating any major extension of the bowel resection. And, incidentally, you will note that my recurrence rate of 30% in cases followed up for 5–18 years is the same as the rate in Bergman and Krause's (1977) more radically treated series followed up for 7–19 years. But in this connection I must mention the recent surprising findings of Papaioannou *et al.* (1979) in Oxford. They surveyed two groups of patients treated by resection for Crohn's disease, in one of which there was histological evidence of disease at the line of resection, whilst, in the other, the ends of the bowel were histologically normal. The incidence of recurrence on follow-up was essentially the same in the two groups.

However, important though recurrence is as a criterion of the success or failure of surgical treatment, it is not everything. At least equally important is the functional or symptomatic state of the patient and his general condition after operation or re-operation. As a measure of that aspect of the outcome of surgery, it is useful to attempt an overall clinical assessment of the results by a system of grading such as that used by Bergman and Krause (1977) and somewhat like the Visick grading that has been employed for many years in judging the comparative results of gastric operations (Goligher *et al.*, 1964). Applying Bergman and Krause's system to my cases at the time of review in 1977/78 gave the results shown in Table 11.3, which incidentally are very similar to Bergman and Krause's own findings.

The patients who were severely handicapped (Category 3) were most often those who had had extensive re-resections. In this connection, I would like to stress that removal of quite considerable amounts of small bowel is often remarkably well tolerated by patients with Crohn's disease because it is frequently effected in stages by re-resection

Table 11.3. *Overall grading of results of resection or re-resection for Crohn's Disease mainly of small bowel at time of review 1978*

Grading of result	Proportion (per cent of 108 cases)
1. VERY GOOD (Virtually no complaints)	79
2. FAIR (Some restriction of capacity for work or leisure because of tiredness or diarrhoea)	15
3. POOR (Severe incapacity on account of diarrhoea, debility or malnutrition)	6

as recurrence takes place, which gives the remaining bowel time to make a functional adaptation. I certainly have four or five patients who have lost half or more of their small gut in this way and yet enjoy good general health with no formidable diarrhoea, partly because they take generous doses of anti-diarrhoeal medication and vitamin B_{12} injections, together with other supplements in some instances. But I can also recall three patients who ended up with more extensive further resections than were originally intended and are now suffering from very serious nutritional deficits. I think the surgeon should always exercise the utmost caution in proceeding to high re-resections of small gut.

Crohn's disease mainly of the large bowel

Though most of the 352 patients mentioned in Table 11.1 with mainly large bowel disease were referred essentially for surgical treatment, many of them were treated medically for a further period before being subjected to operation, and at the time of review in 1977—78, 102 were still being managed conservatively. For most of the 250 (71%) proceeding to surgical treatment this was their first operation, although a few had had previous surgery. And, of course, some of the patients who had their primary or a subsequent operation have undergone further operations for recurrence, so that in the treatment of these 250 patients 326 operations have been employed up to early 1978 (Table 11.4).

Choice of operation

Truelove *et al.* (1965) and Oberhelman *et al.* (1968) suggested that Crohn's colitis might respond better than ordinary ulcerative colitis is known to do (Goligher, 1980) to simple ileostomy, and that the resulting defunctioning of the large bowel might induce the disease in it gradually to resolve, so that the ileostomy could eventually be closed. Unfortunately a subsequent report from Oberhelman and Kohatsu (1971) indicated that this optimistic expectation was seldom realized, and similarly unfavorable experiences with ileostomy (or colostomy) alone were recorded by Jones *et al.* (1966), Burman *et al.* (1971b) and McIlrath (1971). As a consequence, surgical opinion in general is now firmly set in favor of excisional surgery.

Table 11.4. *Operations used in treatment of 225 cases with primary and 79 cases with recurrent Crohn's disease of the large bowel, 1960—78 (from Goligher, 1980)*

Operation employed	For primary disease	For recurrence
Ileostomy + proctocolectomy	124	10
Ileostomy + subtotal colectomy	57	4
Rectal excision	18	0
Colectomy + colo-colonic, ileo-sigmoid or ileo-rectal anastomosis	48	0
Excision of recurrence + ileostomy	0	65
All operations	247	79
Operative deaths	16 (6·5%)	3 (3·8%)

If the lesion is very localized in the colon or rectum, there is no reason why, if surgery should be required, it cannot take the form of a simple segmental colonic resection with colo-colonic anastomosis or an abdomino perineal excision of the rectum with iliac colostomy. But far more frequently the condition is quite extensive and for its surgical removal it is necessary to have recourse to the sort of standard operations that are used in the management of ordinary ulcerative colitis — colectomy and ileorectal anastomosis, and ileostomy with proctocolectomy or subtotal colectomy.

COLECTOMY AND ILEORECTAL ANASTOMOSIS

That pattern of Crohn's colitis, already referred to, in which the rectum and possibly the distal sigmoid are apparently unaffected, would seem *a priori* to be particularly well suited to treatment by colectomy and ileorectal or ileosigmoid anastomosis. In fact 48 (just under 20%) of my large bowel cases coming to surgical treatment were given such anastomoses between 1960 and 1978, sometimes as a primary operation together with a total or subtotal colectomy, sometimes as a primary operation together with a total or subtotal colectomy, sometimes as a secondary procedure after a previous ileostomy and colectomy. There was one operative death; 2 non-fatal anastomotic leaks also occurred. Of 44 patients reviewed in 1978, no less than 26 (59%) had developed recurrent disease – in the ileum proximal to the anastomosis in 15, in the rectum in 7, and in both ileum and rectum in 4. Similar high rates of recurrence have been reported by Baker (1971), Burman *et al.* (1971a), Adson *et al.* (1972), Nugent *et al.* (1973), Lefton *et al.* (1975) and Weterman and Peña (1976). Most of these recurrent cases have needed further operative treatment, usually involving excision of the rectal stump and terminal ileum and conversion to an ileostomy, but some of them have gone for several years with an excellent result before the recurrence appeared. Despite the ultimate poor results of colectomy with ileorectal or ileosigmoid anastomosis, I have little doubt that this operation will continue to be used by many surgeons largely as a means of securing a temporary respite from a permanent ileostomy.

EXCISION WITH ESTABLISHMENT OF A PERMANENT
ILEOSTOMY (OR COLOSTOMY)

The operation commonly favored for the treatment of Crohn's disease affecting mainly or entirely the large bowel has been excision of the affected part with formation of an abdominal stoma, usually by a proctocolectomy or subtotal colectomy with ileostomy, occasionally by an abdominoperineal excision of the rectum with an iliac colostomy. Of my patients, 189 were submitted to this type of operation as the primary surgical procedure, with 16 operative deaths, but in extenuation of this rather high (8%) mortality it should be pointed out that 10 of the fatalities occurred in the group of 34 patients who underwent emergency interventions during severe acute attacks of the disease (Table 11.5). Of the 174 immediate survivors 12 with a retained rectal stump were converted to an ileorectal anastomosis, and 18 died subsequently or were lost to follow-up, leaving 144 traced patients with abdominal stomas, of whom 19 (13·2%) have to date developed recurrences of their disease. In Table 11.6 this incidence of recurrence is contrasted with the overall incidences reported in other similar series of patients. Why there should be such variations from almost nil to nearly 50% is difficult to understand.

All but three of our recurrences were sited just above the stoma, which raises the queries as to whether the original excision had been complete at its upper end and also whether recurrence was more prone to occur in cases where the lower ileum had been involved at the time

Table 11.5. *Immediate results of excision with establishment of an abdominal stoma as primary operation for Crohn's Disease mainly or entirely of large bowel (from Goligher, 1979)*

(a) Operations employed	No. of cases
Ileostomy + proto colectomy	124
Ileostomy + subtotal colectomy	57
A P excision of rectum + colostomy	8
Total operations	189

(b) Results of operations	
*Operative deaths	15
Conversion from ileostomy and subtotal colectomy to ileo-rectal anastomosis	12
Subsequent deaths	
related	4
unrelated	9
Lost to follow-up	5
	45
Patients retaining abdominal stoma available for follow-up	144
No. of patients who have developed recurrence	19 = 13·2%

*N.B. 10 of the operative deaths occurred in 34 patients who underwent operation during severe acute attacks of Crohn's colitis.

of the first operation than when the disease had been confined strictly to the large intestine. Certainly in several of my patients who produced ileal recurrence there were good margins of proximal clearance of the disease in the original operative specimens. As for the influence of ileal involvement, there was no significant difference in the incidence of recurrence whether or not the ileum was implicated originally (Goligher, 1979).

The most important factor influencing the development of recurrent disease appears to be the length of time elapsing since operation (Table

Table 11.6. *Estimates by various authors of the incidence of ileal recurrence after ileostomy and proctocolectomy or subtotal colectomy for Crohn's Disease mainly or entirely of large bowel*

Author	Centre	No. of cases treated	Recurrence (per cent)
Glotzer *et al.* (1970)	Beth Israel Hosp. Boston	?25	?0
Nugent *et al.* (1973)	Lahey Clinic Boston	28	3·3
Ritchie and Lockhart-Mummery (1973)	St Mark's Hosp. London	70	7·1
Steinberg *et al.* (1974)	Birmingham England	65	35·4
Korelitz *et al.* (1972)	Mount Sinai Hosp. N. York City	67	46·0
Goligher (1978)	Leeds Gen. Infirmary England	144 primary opns.	13·2
		70 re-opns.	17·1

11.7). Unfortunately the number of patients available for the follow-up beyond 10 years is relatively small, which impairs the validity of estimates of recurrence after that point, but certainly the impression is of a steadily increasing incidence the longer the follow-up, as has been also observed by Steinberg *et al.* (1974).

In addition to the cases treated primarily under my care by excision and the establishment of an abdominal stoma, there were 79 patients who underwent re-resections for recurrence with the formation of a new stoma. Of these 71 were available for follow-up and the incidence of recurrence after varying periods is shown in Table 11.7, from which it would seem that the development of recurrent disease proceeds at much the same rate as after primary operations.

However, over and above recurrence, there are two other problems that beset the surgical treatment of Crohn's disease of the large bowel. One is that a frequent accompaniment of colectomy or proctocolectomy and ileostomy for this condition is some degree of terminal ile-ectomy, either at the time of the original operation or subsequently to remove disease in the lower ileum. Because of the important absorptive func-

                     J. C. Goligher

Table 11.7. *Frequency of recurrence following resection or re-resection with ileo-stomy (or colostomy) for Crohn's Disease primarily of the large bowel (from Goligher, 1979)*

Type of operation		Length of follow-up in years			
		1–18	5–18	10–18	15–18
Primary resection	No. of cases	144	96	35	14
	No. of recurrences	19 (13%)	17 (18%)	13 (37%)	6 (43%)
Subsequent resection	No. of cases	70	46	27	8
	No. of recurrences	12 (17%)	12 (26%)	9 (33%)	3 (38%)

tion of this part of the small bowel, its loss is apt to result in a profusely acting ileostomy, which can give rise to difficulties in management. However, these can usually be overcome or avoided by the generous use of anti-diarrhoeal agents, such as loperamide, and the regular employment of Stomahesive squares to reinforce the fixation of the ileostomy bag. Incidentally, an additional adverse side-effect of terminal ile-ectomy in these cases, as also in patients with Crohn's disease mainly of the small bowel, is interference with re-absorption of bile acids, resulting in a predisposition to cholelithiasis (Hill *et al.*, 1975).

The other surgical problem relates to the perineal wound, if the rectum has been removed, for its healing is often notoriously delayed in cases of Crohn's disease and may take several months and may require further operative treatment, or even result in a permanent perineal sinus. The management of these difficulties may be extremely tiresome for both patient and surgeon (Goligher, 1980).

Finally, as a small counterblast to the welter of depressing information about the shortcomings of surgical management, there is the overall assessment of the patients' condition at the time of review in 1977–78 (Table 11.8). Of course, no surgeon in his right senses can feel anything like satisfied with the long term results of surgery in the

Table 11.8. *Overall grading of results of resection or re-resection with ileostomy (or colostomy) for Crohn's Disease primarily of large bowel at time of review in 1978*

| | No. of patients in each grade | |
Grading of result	resection (per cent of 119)	re-resection (per cent of 62)
VERY GOOD (virtually no complaints)	81	73
FAIR (some restriction of capacity for work or leisure)	15	19
POOR (Patient severely restricted)	4	8

treatment of Crohn's disease of small or large bowel, but operation often buys time for the patient — and good time at that. Certainly I can recall many patients who had been reduced to an utterly miserable existence before operation, but since have enjoyed many years of symptom-free, full and vigorous life. I have no doubt, therefore, that there is still a major rôle for surgical treatment, despite its defects — at any rate, until such time as the internists are able to turn up some more effective medical treatment than has so far been available. I can hardly wait for that day!

References

Adson M.A., Cooperman A.M. and Farrow G.M. (1972). *Arch. Surg.* **104**, 424.
Atwell J.D., Duthie H.L. and Goligher J.C. (1965) *Brit. J. Surg.* **52**, 996.
Baker W.N.W. (1971) *Gut,* **12**, 427.
Barbour K.W. Jr., Waugh J.M., Beahrs O.H. and Sauer W.G. (1962) *Ann. Surg.* **156**, 472.
Bergman L. and Krause U. (1977) *Scand. J. Gastroenterol.* **12**, 937.
Burman J.H., Cooke W.T. and Williams J.A. (1971a) *Gut,* **12**, 432.
Burman J.H., Williams J.A., Thompson H. and Cooke W.T. (1971b) *Gut,* **12**, 11.
Crohn B.B., Ginsburg L. and Oppenheimer G.D. (1932) *J. Amer. med. Ass.* **99**, 1323.
Garlock J.H., Crohn B.B., Klein S.H. *et al.* (1951) *Gastroenterology,* **19**, 414.

Glotzer D.J., Gardner R.C., Goldman H. *et al.* (1970) *New Engl. J. Med.* **282**, 582.

Goligher J.C. (1979) *Surg. Gynec. Obst.* **148**, 1.

Goligher J.C. (1980) *Surgery of the Anus Rectum and Colon,* 4 e. London: Baillière-Tindall.

Goligher J.C., De Dombal F.T. and Burton I. (1971). In *Progress in Surgery.* Basle: G. Karger.

Goligher J.C., Pulvertaft C.N. and Watkinson G. *et al.* (1964) *Brit. med. J.* i, 455.

Greenstein A.J., Sachar D. and Pucillo A. (1978) *Amer. J. Surg.* **135**, 86.

Hill G.L., Mair W.S.J. and Goligher J.C. (1975) *Gut,* **16**, 932.

Jones J.H., Lennard-Jones J.E. and Lockhart-Mummery H.E. (1966) *Gut,* **7**, 448.

Korelitz B.I., Present D.H., Alpert L.L. *et al.* (1972) *New Engl. J. Med.* **287**, 110.

Koudahl G., Kristensen M. and Lenz K. (1974) *Scand J. Gastroenterol.* **9**, 203.

Krause U., Bergman L. and Norlén B.J. (1971) *Scand. J. Gastroenterol.* **6**, 97.

Lefton H.B., Farmer R.G. and Fazio U. (1975) *Gastroenterology,* **69**, 612.

Lockhart-Mummery H.E. and Morson B.C. (1960) *Gut,* **1**, 87.

Lockhart-Mummery H.E. and Morson B.C. (1964) *Gut,* **5**, 493.

McIlrath D.C. (1971) *Arch. Surg.* **103**, 308.

Nugent F.W., Veidenheimer M.C., Meissner W.A. *et al.* (1973). *Gastroenterology,* **65**, 398.

Oberhelman H.A. Jr., and Kohatsu S. (1971). In *Skandia Symposium on Regional Enteritis (Crohn's Disease).* Stockholm: Nordiska Bokhandelns Förlag.

Oberhelman H.A. Jr., Kohatsu S., Taylor K.B. *et al.* (1968) *Amer. J. Surg.* **115**, 231.

Papaioannou N., Piris J., Lee E.C.G. *et al.* (1979) *Gut,* **20**, A916.

Ritchie J.K. and Lennard-Jones J.E. (1976) *Scand. J. Gastroenterol.* **11**, 433.

Ritchie J.K. and Lockhart-Mummery H.E. (1973) *Gut,* **14**, 263.

Steinberg D.M., Allan R.N., Thompson H. *et al.* (1974) *Gut,* **15**, 845.

Truelove S.C., Ellis H. and Webster C.U. (1965) *Brit. med. J.* i, 150.

van Patter W.N., Bargen J.A., Dockerty M.B. *et al.* (1954) *Gastroenterology,* **26**, 347.

Wenckert A. (1971). In *Skandia Symposium on Regional Enteritis (Crohn's Disease).* Stockholm: Nordiska Bokhandelns Förlag, p. 208.

Weterman I.T. and Peña A.S. (1976) *Scand. J. Gastroenterol,* **11**, 185.

Williams J.A. (1971) *Gut,* **12**, 739.

Young S., Smith I.S., O'Connor J. *et al.* (1975) *Brit. J. Surg.* **62**, 528.

Some Aspects of Ulcerative Colitis

<h1 style="text-align:center">Chapter 12
Aetiology</h1>

D. P. JEWELL

Ulcerative colitis may occur at any age but it is a disease which predominantly presents in young adults. The incidence in the Western World appears to be constant and the disease is now being recognised in most parts of the world. There is a definite familial incidence of around 10% and the affected members may have ulcerative colitis or Crohn's disease (Lewkonia and McConnell, 1976). The factors which render certain individuals and their families susceptible to the disease are, however, unknown. No linkage with common genetic markers, such as blood group or secretor status, has been found and there is no strong association with any of the histo-compatibility antigens apart from those patients who also have ankylosing spondylitis. The majority of these, of course, are positive for HLA-B27. A higher incidence of the disease amongst Jews has been claimed but this may represent an epidemiological problem of population sampling.

Another possible explanation for the familial incidence would be that the disease is caused by an environmental factor. An obvious candidate might be an infection.

The infective theory

When Samuel Wilks described ulcerative colitis in 1859, the major problem was to differentiate it from bacillary dysentery. At first, the disease was thought to be a sequel of dysentery, a view which was strengthened by epidemiological studies reporting ulcerative colitis occurring following outbreaks of dysentery (Felsen and Wolarsky, 1953). A number of organisms were incriminated, such as a diplococcus, *Bacterium necrophorum* and *Serratia marcescens,* but these reports

157

have never been confirmed. More recently, the faecal flora of patients with ulcerative colitis has been shown to be qualitatively similar to the normal flora but the organisms are usually present in greater number (Gorbach *et al.*, 1968). Cooke (1968) has shown that strains of E. coli producing necrotoxins are more common in ulcerative colitis than in healthy individuals. However, these strains tend to appear following a relapse rather than before it.

Cave and his colleagues (1976) have reported the presence of a transmissible agent in colonic tissue from patients with ulcerative colitis in a series of experiments analogous to those in Crohn's disease. The nature of the transmissible agent is not known but the isolation of a small RNA virus has been claimed in a preliminary report. Both of these observations, however, are unconfirmed and, at the present time, there is no strong evidence for a single infective agent as the cause of the disease.

Patients with ulcerative colitis are known to have circulating cytotoxic antibodies to lymphocytes (Strickland *et al.*, 1975) and these lymphocytotoxins are also found more commonly in the relatives of the patients than in the normal population (Korsmeyer *et al.*, 1975). It is not known how they arise but one suggestion is that they are induced by the incorporation of a virus into a lymphocyte or, alternatively, that a viral antigen cross-reacts with an antigen on the lymphocyte surface. Similar antibodies have been found in many other diseases (such as systemic lupus erythematosus, rheumatoid arthritis, infectious mononucleosis and Crohn's disease) and they are, therefore, not specific.

Relatives of patients with ulcerative colitis also show a higher titre of haemagglutinating antibodies to colon than a control population (Lagercrantz *et al.*, 1971). Since these antibodies probably arise by cross-reactivity between colonic and bacterial antigens (Perlmann *et al.*, 1967), it is again possible to argue either that there is a genetic susceptibility to a particular infective agent which is not normally pathogenic or that the disease represents an infection within the community of the family. Against this latter hypothesis, however, is the extreme rarity of inflammatory bowel disease in both husband and wife.

The immunological theory

No single immunological mechanism has emerged to explain the pathogenesis of ulcerative colitis, although many immunological phenomena have been described. They will be summarised by first considering the immune competence of patients with this disease and then considering the types of immune reaction which may contribute to the pathogenesis of the inflammation.

Humoral immunity

The histological picture of ulcerative colitis shows a marked increase of immunoglobulin–producing cells. The greatest increase is in those cells producing IgG but there are also increased numbers of IgA and IgM producing cells (Brandtzaeg *et al.*, 1974; Skinner and Whitehead, 1974). There is little change in serum concentrations of immunoglobulins although they may be mildly elevated in patients with active disease (Hodgson and Jewell, 1978). Metabolic studies have shown increased synthesis and catabolism of IgG and IgM in these patients (Bendixen *et al.*, 1970). With regard to specific antibody, these patients have been reported to have higher titres of antibody to dietary proteins, bacterial antigens and colonic antigens (Taylor and Truelove, 1961; Lagercrantz *et al.*, 1966; Thayer *et al.*, 1969; Brown and Lee, 1974; Wright and Truelove, 1966). It appears, therefore, that these patients are capable of mounting a good immune response to gut-associated antigens although this probably occurs as a result of mucosal inflammation and increased absorption of antigen. However, these raised antibody titres may relate to the fall in circulating suppressor cells which is often associated with active disease (Hodgson *et al.*, 1978).

Cellular immunity

The total lymphocyte counts in these patients are usually within the normal range but there may be a lymphopenia during an acute attack (Strickland *et al.*, 1974).

Similarly, there is little change in the sub-populations of T and B cells. There are contradictory reports of K cell numbers but K cell activity bears no relation to the clinical activity of the disease (Campbell *et al.*, 1976).

Lymphocyte function can be tested using delayed skin hypersensitivity reactions or by assessing the response to non-specific mitogens. Patients with ulcerative colitis show normal responses to antigens such as PPD, Candida, Trichophyton and DNCB which induce a delayed hypersensitivity reaction. Likewise, lymphocytes from these patients transform normally on challenge with PHA and other non-specific mitogens although some authors have reported contrary findings (Thomas and Jewell, 1979).

Immune mechanisms in the pathogenesis of mucosal inflammation

The immune mechanisms that may be playing a role in the pathogenesis of ulcerative colitis will be discussed in relation to the Gell and Coombs classification of immune reactions.

(a) Type I reactions

This type of immune reaction is the immediate hypersensitivity response mediated by IgE antibody. IgE is strongly bound to cells and, in particular, it is bound to mast cells. When antigen binds to specific IgE antibody on a mast cell surface, histamine, kinins, chemotactic factors and a host of other substances are released which result in an inflammatory reaction.

Table 12.1 lists the findings in patients with ulcerative colitis which might support reaginic mechanisms being involved in the pathogenesis of mucosal inflammation. However, definite evidence for such immune responses is weak. Serum IgE concentrations are normal and the positive prick test responses to food allergens are likely to be a secondary phenomenon in the same way that has been suggested for haemagglutinating antibodies to food and bacterial antigens (Mee *et al.*, 1979a). Whether or not there is a genuine increase in atopy in these patients

Table 12.1. *Features suggestive of Type I hypersensitivity*

Eosinophilia in a) peripheral blood
               b) lamina propria

Increased intestinal mast cells.

Positive prick tests to food antigens.

? Increased incidence of atopy.

?? Increase in IgE—producing plasma cells.

---

and their relatives is still not clear, the contradictory results probably representing the difficulties in obtaining satisfactory data for a control population (Mee *et al.*, 1979a). Another field of controversy concerns the number of IgE-producing plasma cells in the inflamed mucosa. In those studies where the specificity of the antisera used has been carefully standardised, no increase in IgE cells has been found (Skinner and Whitehead, 1974; Baklien and Brandtzaeg, 1975). Other studies, however, report quite a marked increase in IgE-producing cells (Heatley *et al.*, 1975a; O'Donoghue and Kumar, 1979). Tissue eosinophils and mast cells are increased in active ulcerative colitis. However, these cells are not specific to Type I reactions and are frequently found in association with Type III reactions.

The initial success obtained with sodium cromoglycate in the treatment of ulcerative colitis tended to support the role of the mast cell in the pathogenesis of the mucosal inflammation (Heatley *et al.*, 1975b; Mani *et al.*, 1976). Subsequent studies employing larger groups of patients, however, have shown little benefit from this drug when used as a maintenance agent (Dronfield and Langman, 1978; Willoughby *et al.*, 1978).

The role of reaginic reactions in the pathogenesis of colonic inflammation must therefore remain *sub judice*.

(b) Type II reactions

This type of reaction involves circulating antibody directed towards cellular antigens and, in the context of human disease, this means an 'auto-antibody'. Auto-antibodies to human colon were first described in children with ulcerative colitis using a haemagglutination technique (Broberger and Perlmann, 1959), but subsequently they have been detected by immunofluorescence (Lagercrantz *et al.*, 1966; Wright and Truelove, 1966).

The antigen is a lipopolysaccharide contained in the goblet cells of the colonic epithelium and it cross-reacts with lipopolysaccharide antigens of colonic bacteria (Perlmann *et al.*, 1967). It seems likely, therefore, that colonic autoantibodies arise in response to immune reactions to colonic bacteria. This is supported by animal experiments in which antibodies to colonic goblet cells have been induced by immunising rabbits with a variety of bacteria (Asherson and Holborrow, 1966; Cooke *et al.*, 1968; Hammarström *et al.*, 1969).

Whether circulating antibodies to colonic epithelium are tissue damaging is unknown but the evidence suggests that they are not. Firstly, only a minority of patients possess these antibodies. Secondly, no relation to any of the clinical features of the disease has been found. Finally, no colonic inflammation has occurred in rabbits in which colonic auto-antibodies have been induced.

(c) Type III reactions

Type III or Arthus reactions are induced by antigen-antibody complexes formed when soluble antigens combine with antibody in the patient's serum or tissue fluid. Large complexes are readily phagocytosed and, if formed in the circulation, they are rapidly cleared by cells of the reticulo-endothelial system. Smaller complexes escape phagocytosis and may circulate in the bloodstream for many hours. Immune complexes cause tissue damage by a variety of mechanisms, some of which are illustrated in Fig. 12.1. Complement activation is one of the major effector mechanisms involved in an Arthus reaction since it releases anaphylatoxins and chemotactants, stimulates release of lysosomal enzymes from a variety of cells, and releases kinins from platelets.

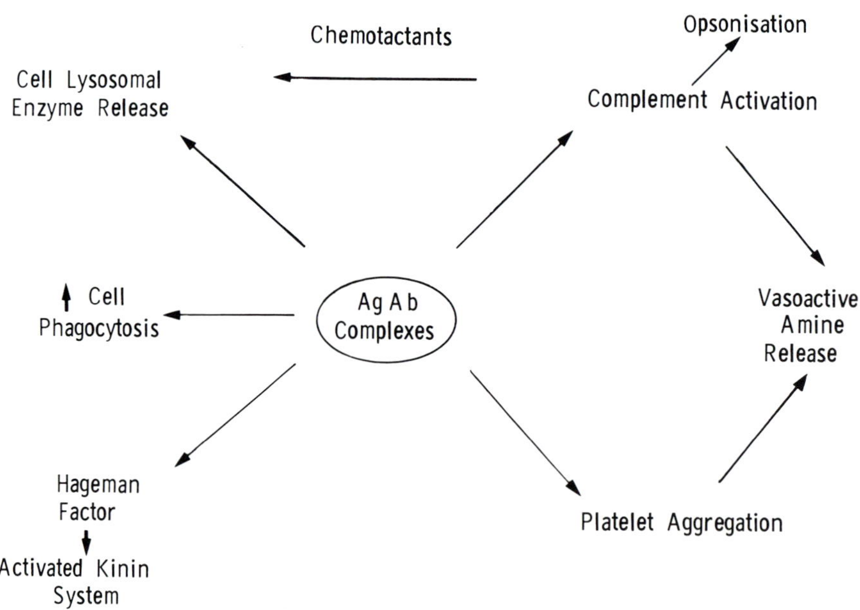

Fig. 12.1. *Mechanisms of tissue damage by immune complexes.*

A wide variety of tests have now been used to detect immune complexes in the sera of patients with ulcerative colitis (Jewell, 1978). These tests have included those which rely on complement fixation, those which detect IgG by Fc binding, and those which determine molecular size. None of them can conclusively prove the presence of immune complexes in serum as opposed to aggregated IgG. Nevertheless, many sera from patients with this disease give positive tests and therefore are thought to contain antigen-antibody complexes or aggregated IgG. These 'complexes' are small (11–18s). They contain IgG and their presence in serum tends to be correlated with activity of the disease and with some of the extra-intestinal manifestations (uveitis, erythema nodosum, acute arthropathy). It is uncommon to find complexes greater than 19s in size, as judged by ^{125}I-Clq binding, but they do occur in patients with associated chronic liver disease (Hodgson *et al.*, 1977a).

Since some of the increased immunoglobulin produced in the inflamed lamina propria has antibody specificity for bacterial antigens (Monteiro *et al.*, 1971), it is reasonable to suppose that antigen-antibody complexes are formed within the colonic mucosa. Direct evidence for this is hard to obtain, since the specificity of immunofluorescent or immunoperoxidase staining is difficult to determine in inflamed tissue. Nevertheless, immunoperoxidase techniques have shown IgG, Clq and C3 in the basement membrane and between the epithelial cells of the colonic mucosa whereas little IgA or IgM was found in these sites (Otto and Gebbers, 1978).

Measurement of serum complement concentrations provides little evidence of complement activation. In fact, C3, Factor B and the modulators of the complement cascade (C$\overline{1}$ INH and C3b INA) behave as acute phase reactants (Hodgson *et al.*, 1977b; Lake *et al.*, 1979; Potter *et al.*, 1980). Since the serum concentration of a protein is the resultant of several factors (e.g. synthesis, catabolism, plasma volume, extravascular distribution), a normal or raised value does not exclude increased metabolism. Direct evidence for complement activation has come from metabolic studies using purified and radio-labelled Clq and C3. For both proteins there is an increase in the synthesis and catabolism in patients with active ulcerative colitis and both proteins sequester in extravascular spaces (Hodgson *et al.*, 1977c; Potter *et al.*, 1979). This latter finding suggests, but does not prove, that complement activation is occurring in the tissues, presumably in the affected colon. A further piece of evidence for complement activation in these patients is the presence of higher titres of immunoconglutinins in their sera than are found in healthy subjects. Immunoconglutinins are antibodies to activated complement components and hence their correlation with the length of history of the colitis suggests continuing complement activation throughout the natural history of the disease (Potter *et al.*, 1980).

It seems very likely, therefore, that immune complex formation with complement activation occurs within the colonic mucosa of patients with ulcerative colitis and that this is one of the major immunological effector mechanisms mediating tissue damage. Immune complexes also release tissue-damaging lysosomal enzymes from cells which may be a further factor in the pathogenesis of the inflammation especially as monocytes contain increased concentrations of these enzymes in patients with active disease (Mee and Jewell, 1980; Mee *et al.*, 1980).

Finally, the importance of Type III reactions in the pathogenesis of ulcerative colitis is supported by the close similarity between the histological features of the disease and the features of an Arthus reaction, namely, increased vascularity and an acute inflammatory infiltrate of neutrophils, eosinophils and plasma cells.

(d) Type IV reactions

These immunological reactions rely on cell-mediated immunity and involve sensitised T lymphocytes. Cellular hypersensitivity can be detected by delayed skin test responses (eg. the Mantoux test) or by *in vitro* tests such as lymphocyte transformation and leucocyte migration inhibition.

In ulcerative colitis, evidence for cell-mediated hypersensitivity is confusing and will not be reviewed in detail. Fink and Mais (1968) reported positive delayed skin tests to a suspension of autologous colon but only when the colonic suspension had been previously incubated with live E. coli. Further evidence for cellular hypersensitivity to bacterial and colonic antigens has come from experiments utilising lymphocyte transformation and leucocyte migration inhibition tests. Unfortunately not everyone has been able to reproduce these results but, on balance, the evidence is in favour of T cell sensitisation to these antigens (Thomas and Jewell, 1979).

(e) Lymphocyte cytotoxicity

Perlmann and Broberger (1963) were the first to show that peripheral blood white cells from patients with ulcerative colitis were able to kill colonic epithelial cells. These observations have been extended by Shorter and his colleagues and are summarised in Table 12.2. The phenomenon appears specific for ulcerative colitis and Crohn's disease, and lymphocytes from all such patients have this facility. The nature of the effector lymphocyte is not known, although it appears to be a cell bearing an Fc receptor but without T or B cell markers (Stobo *et al.*, 1975). The exact immunological mechanisms involved in the reaction, its inhibition by bacteria and serum factors and its induction in normal lymphocytes are quite obscure. Nevertheless, epithelial cell destruction by lymphocytes could play a major role in the inflammatory response. Perhaps it is noteworthy, however, that it is neutrophils rather than lymphocytes that are seen passing between the epithelial cells and causing destruction of the glands.

Discussion

Several immunological reactions may therefore contribute to the pathogenesis of ulcerative colitis and more than one type of immune response may be required before the disease develops. Throughout this chapter, immune responses to bacteria have been prominent. Bacterial antigens will induce antibody which cross-reacts with colonic epithelium, specific antibody to bacteria is synthesised locally in the mucosa, there may be

Table 12.2. *Lymphocytotoxicity in ulcerative colitis*

1 Only present in ulcerative colitis and Crohn's disease.

2 May be abolished by colectomy but persists during remission.

3 Specific for colonic epithelium.

4 Does not require complement.

5 Inhibited by:
   a) Sera from other patients with inflammatory bowel disease.
   b) lipopolysaccharide extract of E. coli.

6 Induced in normal lymphocytes by:
   a) sera from patients with inflammatory bowel disease.
   b) lipopolysaccharide extract of E. coli.

lymphocytes sensitised to bacterial antigens in the peripheral blood and bacteria can influence the lymphocytotoxic reaction. It is certainly possible, therefore, that ulcerative colitis develops when some or all of these responses occur simultaneously.

Further evidence incriminating immune responses to bacteria comes from animal studies. As previously mentioned, the presence of circulating auto-antibodies to colonic epithelium, induced by immunisation of rabbits with bacteria, does not cause colonic inflammation. However, prior sensitisation to bacterial antigens does affect the development of colonic inflammation if the colon is damaged by other mechanisms. Intravenous injection of soluble immune complexes into rabbits who have suffered mild irritation of the rectum causes an acute colitis which heals by six weeks. If, on the other hand, this experiment is repeated with animals possessing high circulating antibody titres to bacterial antigens then a chronic colitis develops which is still present six months after the injection of immune complexes (Mee *et al.*, 1979b). The histological features of this experimental lesion are closely similar to those of the human disease. These findings support the role of antigen-antibody complexes in the pathogenesis of ulcerative colitis and suggest that chronicity may depend on previous immunisation with gut-associated antigens (colonic, bacterial or dietary). Nevertheless, a similar histological picture can also be produced experimentally by sensitising the colon with DNCB (Rabin and Rogers, 1978). In other words, features of a typical Arthus reaction in the colon do not necessarily indicate a Type III reaction but may also be produced by cell-mediated mechanisms.

The hypothesis that chronic ulcerative colitis may be largely due to a variety of immune responses to gut-associated antigens is an attractive one. The immune-complex rabbit model may also provide insight into one mechanism whereby relapses occur since circulating complexes can presumably deposit in a damaged human colon as they can in a rabbit colon. This would provide a good explanation for the observation that patients with ulcerative colitis have a high risk of relapsing if they develop a minor infection (Mee and Jewell, 1978). Perhaps the major challenge to our understanding of the aetiology of the disease is its anatomical distribution. So far, there are no clues to explain why the disease begins in the rectum and why it is confined to the colon. Subtle changes in the bacterial flora or in the metabolism of colonic epithelial cells in different parts of the colon (Roediger, 1979) may be relevant.

References

Asherson G.L. and Holborrow E.J. (1966) *Immunology*, **10**, 161.

Baklien K. and Brandtzaeg P. (1975) *Clin. exp. Immunol.* **22**, 197.

Bendixon G., Goltermann N., Jarnum S., Jensen K.B., Weeke B. and Westergaard H. (1970) *Scand. J. Gastroenterol.* **5**, 433.

Brandtzaeg P., Baklien K., Fausa O. and Hoel P.S. (1974) *Gastroenterology*, **66**, 1123.

Broberger O. and Perlmann P. (1959) *J. exp. Med.* **110**, 657.

Brown W.R. and Lee E. (1974) *Gastroenterology*, **66**, 1145.

Campbell A.C., Nunne J.M., MacLennan I.C.M., Waller C.A., Wood J., Jewell D.P. and Truelove S.C. (1976) *Clin. exp. Immunol.* **24**, 249.

Cave D.R., Mitchell D.N. and Brooke B.N. (1976) *Lancet*, i, 1311.

Cooke E.M. (1968) *J. Path. Bact.* **95**, 101.

Cooke E.M., Filipe M.I. and Dawson I.M.P. (1968) *J. Path. Bact.* **96**, 125.

Dronfield M.W. and Langman M.J.S. (1978) *Gut*, **19**, 1136.

Felsen J. and Wolarsky W. (1953) *J. Amer. med. Ass.* **153**, 1069.

Fink S. and Mais R.F. (1968) *Gut*, **9**, 629.

Gorbach S.L., Nahas L., Plaut A.G., Weinstein L., Patterson J.E. and Levitan R. (1968) *Gastroenterology*, **54**, 575.

Hammarström S., Perlmann P., Gustafsson B.E. and Lagercrantz R. (1969) *J. exp. Med.* **129**, 747.

Heatley R.V., Rhodes J., Calcraft B.J., Whitehead R.H., Fifield R. and Newcombe R.G. (1975a) *Lancet*, ii, 1010.

Heatley R.V., Calcraft B.J., Rhodes J., Owen E. and Evans B.K. (1975b) *Gut*, **16**, 559.

Hodgson H.J.F. and Jewell D.P. (1978) *Amer. J. dig. Dis.* **23**, 123.

Hodgson H.J.F., Potter B.J. and Jewell D.P. (1977a) *Clin. exp. Immunol.* **29**, 187.

Hodgson H.J.F., Potter B.J. and Jewell D.P. (1977b) *Gut*, **18**, 749.

Hodgson H.J.F., Potter B.J. and Jewell D.P. (1977c) *Clin. exp. Immunol.* **28**, 490.

Hodgson H.J.F., Wands J.R. and Isselbacher K.J. (1978) *Clin. exp. Immunol.* **32**, 451.

Jewell D.P. (1978). In *Topics in Gastroenterology*, p. 311, ed. Truelove S.C. and Heyworth M.F. Blackwell Scientific Publications.

Korsmeyer S.J., Williams R.C., Wilson I.D. and Strickland R.G. (1975) *New Engl. J. Med.* **293**, 1117.

Lagercrantz R., Perlmann P. and Hammarström S. (1971) *Gastroenterology*, **60**, 381.

Lagercrantz R., Hammarström S., Perlmann P. and Gustafsson B.E. (1966) *Clin. exp. Immunol.* **1**, 263.

Lake A.M., Stitzel A.E., Urmson J.R., Walker W.A. and Spitzer R.E. (1979) *Gastroenterology*, **76**, 1374.

Lewkonia R.M. and McConnell R.B. (1976) *Gut*, **17**, 235.

Mani V., Green F.H.Y., Lloyd G., Fox H. and Turnberg L.A. (1976) *Lancet*, i, 439.

Mee A.S. and Jewell D.P. (1978) *Brit. med. J.* iii, 801.

Mee A.S. and Jewell D.P. (1980) *Clin. Sci.* **58**, 295.

Mee A.S., Brown D. and Jewell D.P. (1979a) *Scand. J. Gastroenterol.* **14**, 743.

Mee A.S., McLaughlin J.E., Hodgson H.J.F. and Jewell D.P. (1979b) *Gut,* **20,** 1.

Mee A.S., Nuttall L., Potter B.J. and Jewell D.P. (1980) *Clin. exp. Immunol.* **39,** 785.

Monteiro E., Fossey J., Shiner M., Drasar B.S. and Allison A.C. (1971) *Lancet,* i, 249.

O'Donoghue D.P. and Kumar P. (1979) *Gut,* **20,** 149.

Otto H.F. and Gebbers J.-O. (1978) *Inn. Med.* **2,** 69.

Perlmann P. and Broberger O. (1963) *J. Exp. Med.* **117,** 717.

Perlman P., Hammarström S., Lagercrantz R. and Campbell D. (1967) *Proc. Soc. exp. Biol.* (N.Y.) **125,** 975.

Potter B.J., Hodgson H.J.F., Mee A.S. and Jewell D.P. (1979) *Gut,* **20,** 1012.

Potter B.J., Brown D.J.C., Watson A. and Jewell D.P. (1980) *Gut* (in press).

Rabin B.S. and Rogers S.J. (1978) *Gastroenterology,* **75,** 29.

Roediger W.E.W. (1979). In *Topics in Gastroenterology 7,* p. 281 ed. Truelove S.C. and Willoughby C.P. Blackwell Scientific Publications.

Skinner J.M. and Whitehead R. (1974) *J. clin. Path.* **27,** 643.

Stobo J.D., Tomasi T.B., Huizenga K.A., Spencer R.J. and Shorter R.G. (1976) *Gastroenterology,* **70,** 171.

Strickland R.G., Korsmeyer S., Soltis R.D., Wilson I.D. and Williams R.C. (1974) *Gastroenterology,* **67,** 569.

Strickland R.G., Friedler E.M., Henderson C.A., Wilson I.D. and Williams R.C. (1975) *Clin. exp. Immunol.* **21,** 384.

Taylor K.B. and Truelove S.C. (1961) *Brit. med. J.* ii, 924.

Thayer W.R., Brown M., Sangree M.H., Katz J. and Hersch T. (1969) *Gastroenterology,* **57,** 311.

Thomas H.C. and Jewell D.P. (1979) *'Clinical Gastrointestinal Immunology'* Chap. 10. Blackwell Scientific Publications.

Willoughby C.P., Piris J., Heyworth M. and Truelove S.C. (1979) *Lancet,* i, 119.

Wright R. and Truelove S.C. (1966) *Gut,* **7,** 32.

Chapter 13
Ulcerative colitis beginning
in childhood

S. C. TRUELOVE

It is generally agreed that ulcerative colitis beginning in childhood often runs a severe course. Until fairly recently, the prognosis was bad. For example, Devroede *et al.* (1971) made an important study of the outcome in 396 children with ulcerative colitis seen at the Mayo Clinic from 1919 to 1965. Follow-up information was complete for 70% and partial for another 10%. Actuarial methods were used in the analysis of the data. They reached the following main conclusions:

1. The death rate was 20% per decade.
2. The risk of developing cancer of the large bowel was 20% per decade after the first decade of ulcerative colitis.
3. The risk of death and of cancer was particularly high when the entire colon was involved.
4. Proctocolectomy improved the prognosis.

Devroede *et al.* also found no improvement in the survival of patients after 1953, suggesting that the introduction of corticosteroids had not appreciably affected the prognosis.

Hijmans and Enzer (1962) reported on the outcome in 43 patients seen at Duke University Hospital between 1932 and 1960. In two-thirds of the patients, the disease ran a severe course. There were seven deaths (16.3%) during a short period of follow-up. Four of these deaths occurred after emergency surgery and it seems likely that this was because the surgery was often delayed and was only employed 'in dire emergency', to use the authors' own words. There were no cases of cancer of the large bowel but the follow-up period was short.

Korelitz *et al.* (1962) reported the results in 84 children at the Mount Sinai Hospital, New York, between 1929 and 1958. In the 'pre-steroid' era, 85% of the patients suffered from complications of the disease, including 10% who developed cancer. The mortality was formidable, 43% of the patients having died directly or indirectly from the ulcerative colitis. They commented that 'at least half the deaths following operation are caused in part by late intervention when surgery is poorly tolerated'. In a separate article, Korelitz and Gribetz (1962) covered the results in the post-steroid era. They found that the frequency of complications of the disease was unchanged but that the overall mortality was lower, possibly because elective surgery was more widely used.

Recent surveys

Much more favourable results have been obtained when children with ulcerative colitis have been treated along the same lines as those that have been developed for adults. This implies three things:

1. Intensive medical therapy for severe attacks with rapid resort to emergency colectomy if the response is not good.
2. Elective surgery when chronic disease is not well controlled by medical treatment.
3. Prophylactic proctocolectomy in patients with universal colitis of more than 10 years duration in order to eliminate the risk of cancer of the large bowel.

Werlin and Grand (1977) reported on the outcome of severe ulcerative colitis in 14 children and adolescents. Intensive medical treatment induced remission within 12 days in four patients, but further medical treatment produced little improvement in the remainder. Seven of these patients were treated by colectomy during the acute phase of the disease and elective colectomy was performed in some others during the course of follow-up. There were no deaths and the authors make the comment that 'although medical treatment must be vigorous, it must not be prolonged . . . we believe that the current practice of prolonged medical treatment for severe colitis needs to be revised.'

From Denmark, Binder *et al.* (1973) have reported on 62 patients treated during the period 1961—71, in whom colectomy had been performed in 46% after eight years of observation. The mortality was only 3% for the entire group and no cases of cancer of the colon were encountered.

Personal series

In 1973, I reported the results of a personal series of patients with ulcerative colitis beginning in childhood dealt with during the 10-year period 1963–72 (Truelove, 1973). The following patients were excluded:

1. Patients with disease confined to the rectum (haemorrhagic proctitis) as this condition usually runs a more benign course than more extensive colitis.
2. Patients referred to me simply for a second opinion.

After these exclusions, there were 57 patients, all with classical ulcerative colitis and all of whom I treated for the whole, or at least a substantial part, of the period under review. The mean period of surveillance was more than six years and at that time only one patient had died (after proctocolectomy) and all the others were living normal lives, albeit under medical supervision. At that time, 9 of the 57 patients had been treated by proctocolectomy (with one death, as already mentioned) and there had been one case of cancer of the colon apparently cured by proctocolectomy (Table 13.1).

Present state of the patients

For the purpose of the present chapter, I have attempted to get up-to-date information on all these 57 patients. Many are still attending our Ulcerative Colitis Clinic at Oxford but others, not surprisingly, have moved away and in some of these the follow-up information is incom-

Table 13.1. *Results in 57 patients with ulcerative colitis beginning in childhood at two different stages of follow-up*

	Mean period of follow-up in years	
	6 years	12 years
Deaths	1 (1.8%)	3 (5.3%)
Proctocolectomy	9* (15.8%)	16* (28.1%)
Living normally without operation	48 (84.2%)	39 (68.4%)

*includes 1 death

plete. However, the minimum period of follow-up is seven years and the mean period of follow-up is just over 12 years.

Deaths

The number of deaths has increased to three and their details are as follows:

1. A boy developed universal colitis at the age of seven years. He was treated with corticosteroids for a year in another hospital before being transferred to Oxford, by which time he was severely hypercorticoid and had bilateral renal calculi. After a while he was taken out of my care by his parents and was treated by proctocolectomy in a London teaching hospital but he died postoperatively. The main error in this case was continuation of corticosteroid therapy in the face of persistent symptoms; he should have been treated by proctocolectomy much earlier in the course of the illness. (This was the one death in the series reported by me in 1973).

2. A boy developed universal colitis at the age of seven years and this was complicated by chronic liver disease. When he came under my care, he already had pronounced splenomegaly and other evidence of portal hypertension. The colitis was comparatively mild and required little treatment. He suffered from episodes of haematemesis and he was treated by a portacaval shunt at the age of 18 years. However, when aged 20 years, he died in another hospital after a massive haematemesis.

3. A girl developed universal colitis at the age of seven years. The illness pursued a typical intermittent course, but she responded well to medical treatment for 12 years while attending our clinic. She then married and moved away. She returned to the clinic subsequently on a single occasion, when she was ill with colitic symptoms and with sigmoido-scopic evidence of severe active colitis. She refused treatment and did not attend again, but she subsequently died (details of the death unknown).

Cancer of the colon

There has been only a single case, which was reported in 1973. The patient was a boy who developed ulcerative colitis at the age of seven years. When he was aged 14, I advised proctocolectomy but this was refused and his parents stopped bringing him to our clinic. When he was 17, he was admitted to another hospital with severe symptoms of ulcerative colitis and was treated by proctocolectomy. The operation specimen revealed that he had a carcinoma of the ascending colon with involvement of the regional lymph nodes. However, he is still perfectly well 10 years after the operation.

Proctocolectomy

As already mentioned, nine of these patients had already been treated by proctocolectomy by 1973, with one death. A further seven patients have been similarly treated during the succeeding period of follow-up, making a total of 16 patients (28% of the series). There have been no further deaths among the patients treated and the 15 survivors are all living normal lives. With the exception of the patient who died and the one who was found at proctocolectomy to have a cancer of the colon, all these operations were performed by my surgical colleagues in Oxford.

Patients treated medically

Even though a substantial proportion of the patients have been treated by proctocolectomy, the majority have continued to be managed medically with satisfactory results. The 39 patients in this category were all living normal lives at the end of follow-up although it must be expected that some of them may require to be treated by proctocolectomy in the future. Of these 39 patients, 20 were on maintenance therapy with sulphasalazine but 19 were in prolonged remission while receiving no treatment.

Marriage and children

Some notion of the capacity of the patients to lead normal lives can be gleaned from considering the marital status of the female members of the series. Of the 35 girls in the series, 12 are not married but some of these are still very young and are likely to marry in the future. Of the 23 who have married, 16 have borne children and the size of their families appears to approximate to what is usual in our society, as the children range in number from one to five, with two or three being the usual figure. Some of the seven married women without children have been married fairly recently and have not yet decided to start a family.

                                    S. C. Truelove

Overall results

A simple view of the overall results in the present series is given in
Table 13.1.

Comparison with other series

Although the results of the present study show that ulcerative colitis
beginning in childhood is still a dangerous disease, it also indicates that
the outcome is much more favourable nowadays than it was formerly.
For example, if the experience of the Mayo Clinic up to 1965 (Devroede
et al., 1971) had been duplicated in the Oxford series, there would have
been 14 deaths among the 57 patients instead of the three that have
actually occurred. As it is, our results correspond fairly closely to those
published by Binder *et al.* (1973) for a series of children dealt with at
roughly the same time as the present series and in roughly the same way.

Subsequent experience

This chapter has described the outcome to date of 57 patients with
ulcerative colitis beginning in childhood who attended the Ulcerative
Colitis Clinic in Oxford during the period 1963–72. This was a period
when the medical and surgical treatment of ulcerative colitis was in
a stage of development. The method of treating a severe attack of
ulcerative colitis by a short period of intensive medical treatment with
resort to emergency colectomy if there is not a rapid favourable response
was in process of evolution among our adult cases and has led to the
situation in which death in an acute attack has been virtually eliminated
(Truelove and Jewell, 1974; Truelove *et al.*, 1978). At the same time
we were learning to treat children with the disease along exactly the
same lines as those that worked best with the adult patients. The
benefit of this approach has been reflected in our more recent
experience. Since 1972, a number of other children with ulcerative
colitis have been dealt with and there have been no deaths among them,
although several have required to be treated by proctocolectomy, sometimes as an emergency procedure. In effect, it is my belief that the
application of modern medical and surgical methods to the treatment
of ulcerative colitis in childhood has resulted in a substantial improvement in the outcome.

Conclusions

Ulcerative colitis beginning in childhood often affects the entire colon and frequently runs a severe course. In the past, it was a very dangerous disease with a high fatality rate. To obtain good results, it is essential to treat children with the disease along precisely the same lines as adults. This implies intensive medical treatment for any severe attack with resort to emergency colectomy if there is not a rapid response. Elective proctocolectomy is required for chronic disease not responding well to medical treatment. Prophylactic proctocolectomy is required in some patients when the disease has been present for more than 10 years to eliminate the risk of cancer of the colon.

References

Binder V., Bonnevie O., Gertz T.Cl., Krasilnikoff P.A., Vestermark S. and Riis P. (1973) *Scand. J. Gastroenterol.* 8, 161.

Devroede G.J., Taylor W.F., Sauer W.G., Jackman R.J. and Stickler G.B. (1971) *New Engl. J. Med.* 285, 17.

Hijmans J.C. and Enzer N.B. (1962) *Pediatrics,* 29, 389.

Korelitz B.I., Gribetz D. and Danziger I. (1962) *Ann. intern. Med.* 57, 582.

Korelitz B.I. and Gribetz D. (1962) *Ann. intern. Med.* 57, 592.

Truelove S.C. (1973) *Proc. roy. Soc. Med.* 66, 1032.

Truelove S.C. and Jewell D.P. (1974) *Lancet,* i, 1067.

Truelove S.C., Willoughby C.P., Lee E.G. and Kettlewell M.G.W. (1978) *Lancet,* ii, 1086.

Werlin S.L. and Grand R.J. (1977) *Gastroenterology,* 73, 828.

Chapter 14
Ulcerative colitis and pregnancy

C. P. WILLOUGHBY

Ulcerative colitis commonly begins in adolescence or early adult life and therefore frequently coexists with the active reproductive years of the women who develop the disease. An association between the onset of ulcerative colitis and pregnancy or the puerperium was first mentioned by Gossage and Price (1909), but these authors did not provide details of the course of the disease in their patients. The general experience in various small series of cases reported during the first half of the century was that pregnancy had an adverse effect on ulcerative colitis, and that maternal deaths were not uncommon (Abramson *et al.*, 1951). More recent studies have implied a rather better outlook both for the pregnancy and the colitis (Crohn *et al.*, 1956; MacDougall, 1956; Banks *et al.*, 1957; de Dombal *et al.*, 1965; McEwan, 1972; Webb and Sedlack, 1974). However, all these studies were retrospective and were largely based on information relating to patients who did not receive modern medical treatment; there has been no major survey for the past 15 years, during which time various developments in medical therapy have occurred.

We have just finished collecting data on patients who attended the ulcerative colitis clinic at the Radcliffe Infirmary and the John Radcliffe Hospital, Oxford, during the 20-year period 1960–1979 inclusive. The analysis of the data is not yet complete, but some of the interim results will be incorporated in this Chapter. The full results will be published elsewhere (Willoughby and Truelove, 1980).

Ulcerative colitis and fertility

It is usually stated that fertility is normal in women with ulcerative colitis. Crohn *et al.* (1956) considered that fertility was not affected by the disease in the patients whom they surveyed but they did not provide detailed figures to confirm this. MacDougall (1956) recorded that, out of 131 women of childbearing age, 64 (49%) were pregnant when their colitis first started, or became pregnant at some time after the disease had been diagnosed. Banks *et al.* (1957) found that 56 out of 133 women in their series (42%) became pregnant, but they did not mention the proportion of the women in the study who were premenopausal. In the survey of de Dombal *et al.* (1965), out of 229 women who suffered from ulcerative colitis while of an age to bear children, 72 (31%) became pregnant, but this was obviously an underestimate of the true fertility rate, as the follow-up period was short.

In our present study, of the 147 women patients who had not completed their families before the ulcerative colitis began, 119 (81%) have been pregnant since the disease was diagnosed or, in nine cases, immediately before its onset. 28 women have not conceived, and in 18 of these infertility is voluntary. Only ten women have been unable to have children, representing 6·8% of the 147 women potentially able to do so. This compares favourably with the estimate that 10% of all marriages in this country are childless because of fertility problems (Harrison, 1977).

It is interesting to note, that, of the 18 cases of voluntary infertility, three women had deliberately avoided having children because of medical advice from other clinicians that pregnancy was likely to have an adverse effect on the course of their ulcerative colitis. Such advice was frequently given to patients before the advent of specific medical therapy for the disease (Kleckner *et al.*, 1951), but current data show that the prognosis for both pregnancy and colitis is now very much more favourable than was once the case.

Ulcerative colitis and the outcome of pregnancy

Most previous series indicate that ulcerative colitis has no adverse effect on the outcome of pregnancy. Table 14.1 shows the overall results in our current study compared with those from earlier surveys and with figures for the general population in England and Wales. The outcome of the 172 pregnancies in our series which did not end in abortion is shown in Table 14.2.

It can be seen that the outcome of pregnancy is very similar to that

Table 14.1. *Effect of ulcerative colitis on the outcome of pregnancy*

Survey	Number of pregnancies	Normal live births	Spontaneous abortion	Therapeutic abortion	Congenital abnormality	Stillbirth
Abramson *et al.* (1951)	46	36	3	6	0	1
Kleckner *et al.* (1951)	19	17	2	0	0	0
Crohn *et al.* (1956)	150	125	12	8	0	5
MacDougall (1956)	100	80	13	4	0	3
Banks *et al.* (1957)	78	63	3	9	1	2
de Dombal *et al.* (1965)	107	90	7	5	3	2
McEwan (1972)	50	44	4	1	0	1
Webb and Sedlack (1974)	79	60	13	3	2	1
Total	629	515 (82%)	57 (9%)	36 (6%)	6 (1%)	15 (2%)
Oxford series (1980)	204	165 (81%)	23 (11%)	9 (5%)	5 (2%)	2 (1%)
Normal population* (1977)		77%	12%	8%	2%	1%

*Derived from reports of the Office of Population Censuses and Surveys. (Spontaneous abortion rate assumed to be 12% – see Stevenson *et al.*, 1959).

Table 14.2. *Analysis of 172 births to women with ulcerative colitis. The figures for the normal population are from Donald (1974)*

		Ulcerative colitis patients		Normal population
Infant	Full term	144	(84%)	
	Low birth weight	16	(9%)	4–10%
	Postmature	10	(6%)	2%
	Stillbirth	2	(1%)	1%
Delivery	Normal	132	(77%)	
	Instrumental	31	(18%)	10–14%
	Caesarean section	9	(5%)	1– 8%

expected in normal women, and further analysis of our data shows that the chance of a normal live baby is particularly high for those patients whose ulcerative colitis is in remission when they become pregnant. Patients whose colitis is active at the time of conception have a slightly less favourable prognosis as far as the result of the pregnancy is concerned. In particular, the incidence of therapeutic abortion in these patients is about three times that in patients whose colitis was in remission at the start of pregnancy, the risk of a premature baby is approximately doubled, and the two stillbirths in the series also occurred in this group.

Sixteen women developed ulcerative colitis for the first time during a pregnancy; in 14 of these pregnancies a normal live baby resulted (although two were born prematurely) and two spontaneous abortions occurred. All nine women whose ulcerative colitis started in the puerperium had normal live births before the onset of their disease.

The effect of pregnancy on ulcerative colitis

In the past it was considered that ulcerative colitis beginning during or shortly after pregnancy was liable to run a particularly severe course (Abramson *et al.*, 1951; Zetzel, 1954; Crohn *et al.*, 1956; MacDougall, 1956; Banks *et al.*, 1957). The behaviour of an established case of colitis during pregnancy and the puerperium depends to some extent on its state of activity at the time of conception. It has become conventional to discuss the effects of pregnancy on ulcerative colitis in terms of the four categories of patients originally described by Abramson *et al.* (1951):

(1) Patients whose ulcerative colitis is in remission at the time of conception
(2) Patients with active ulcerative colitis at the start of pregnancy
(3) Patients who develop ulcerative colitis during pregnancy
(4) Patients whose ulcerative colitis begins in the puerperium (within three months of childbirth)

1. Patients in remission at the time of conception

Patients whose ulcerative colitis is quiescent when they conceive have a good chance of remaining symptom-free throughout their pregnancy (Table 14.3). We have found that only 30% are liable to relapse in pregnancy or the puerperium. This is probably not much higher than would be expected for a similar non-pregnant group of patients with ulcerative colitis followed up for one year.

Relapses of quiescent ulcerative colitis have been found to occur predominantly in the first trimester of pregnancy and in the puerperium (Crohn *et al.*, 1956; de Dombal *et al.*, 1965, McEwan, 1972). Whether the risk of recurrence reflects changes in the circulating endogenous corticosteroid levels at these times is uncertain (Crohn *et al.*, 1956; de Dombal *et al.*, 1965). In our patients, 17 out of the 37 relapses

Table 14.3. *Course of ulcerative colitis in remission at the start of pregnancy*

Survey	Number of pregnancies	Remission maintained	Relapse in pregnancy or puerperium
Abramson *et al.* (1951)	20	13	7 (35%)
Crohn *et al.* (1956)	74	34	40 (54%)
MacDougall (1956)	21	19	2 (10%)
Banks *et al.* (1957)	46	33	13 (28%)
de Dombal *et al.* (1965)	80	53	27 (34%)
McEwan (1972)	25	21	4 (16%)
Total	266	173 (65%)	93 (35%)
Oxford series (1980)	124	87 (70%)	37 (30%)

occurred in the first three months of pregnancy, but the remainder were divided equally among the other trimesters and the puerperium. Therefore, an excessive liability to relapse after delivery has not been confirmed for this group of patients.

2. Patients with active ulcerative colitis at the start of pregnancy

Patients in this group generally do less well than those whose disease is quiescent at the time of conception (Table 14.4). The general experience has been that almost half of them deteriorate during or shortly after pregnancy, but in our recent series only one-third of the patients actually became worse. Nevertheless, only a minority improved and 60% of the group continued to have symptoms throughout their pregnancy and in the puerperium.

In all previous series, the risk of deterioration was highest in the first trimester and in the puerperium, and the disease frequently became severe. Abramson and his colleagues (1951) found that therapeutic abortion usually resulted in a rapid remission of symptoms and they recommended that pregnancy should be terminated in all cases where a severe attack developed in the first trimester. This view was shared by Crohn *et al.* (1956), but they commented that the effect of cortico-steroids in checking attacks of the disease might reduce the necessity for therapeutic abortion. Subsequent experience suggests that termination

Table 14.4. *Course of ulcerative colitis in patients with active disease at the start of pregnancy*

Survey	Number of pregnancies	Improved	Unchanged	Worse during pregnancy or puerperium
Abramson *et al.* (1951)	17	0	0	17 (100%)
Crohn *et al.* (1956)	38	–	–	29 (76%)
MacDougall (1956)	53	25	15	13 (25%)
Banks *et al.* (1957)	23	3	13	7 (30%)
de Dombal *et al.* (1965)	3	2	1	0 (0%)
McEwan (1972)	22	8	4	10 (45%)
Total	156	38	33	76 (49%)
Oxford series (1980)	55	22	15	18 (33%)

of pregnancy may not, by itself, improve many of the patients who have severe relapses of colitis (de Dombal *et al.*, 1965). We have found that active ulcerative colitis during pregnancy usually responds to standard medical therapy with sulphasalazine and corticosteroids, and we have not ourselves recommended therapeutic abortion as part of the management of any patient. Four patients in our series did have terminations on medical advice from other clinicians, but it is questionable whether the intervention improved the course of their disease: two of them, who also received systemic corticosteroids, improved; one was unchanged; and one continued to deteriorate and came to emergency colectomy a week later.

3. Ulcerative colitis beginning during pregnancy

In previous studies, this group of patients has had the worst outlook. Abramson *et al.* (1951) reported five women in this category, four of whom died shortly after delivery. Crohn *et al.* (1956) had one maternal death in 19 pregnancies. The colitis most frequently starts early in pregnancy (Crohn *et al.*, 1956) and severe first attacks are said to be common (Abramson *et al.*, 1951; Crohn *et al.*, 1956; MacDougall, 1956). The long-term prognosis of such patients was found to be poor by Banks *et al.* (1957), repeated relapses of the disease eventually leading to death in two out of five patients in the group.

During the last 20 years, 16 of our patients have had their first attacks of ulcerative colitis while pregnant. Eight of these were in the first trimester and seven in the second trimester of pregnancy. Only four of the attacks were severe, three of which occurred in early pregnancy, and all were easily controlled by standard medical treatment. There were no maternal deaths in this group, or in the rest of the series, so it is probable that modern methods of therapy have greatly reduced the risk to the mother's life.

4. Onset of ulcerative colitis in the puerperium

Ulcerative colitis beginning in the puerperium is also said to be particularly hazardous, as severe attacks were common in previous series and there was an appreciable risk (about 13%) of maternal death (Abramson *et al.*, 1951; Crohn *et al.*, 1956; MacDougall, 1956; Banks *et al.*, 1957). This is in contrast to our own recent experience. In our series, there were nine patients in this category; in eight of them the initial attack of colitis was mild, and in the other it was only moderately severe.

Ulcerative colitis in successive pregnancies

Crohn and his colleagues (1956) suggested that women who had severely active ulcerative colitis during a pregnancy should be advised not to have further children. However, both MacDougall (1956) and McEwan (1972) found that the course of colitis during one pregnancy did not predict the behaviour of the disease in subsequent pregnancies. Our experience is similar. Sixty two of our patients had more than one pregnancy after the onset of ulcerative colitis. In 29 of them (47%) the colitis has always been unaffected by pregnancy, while ten patients (16%) consistently became worse. However, 23 of the women (37%) showed an inconsistent reaction, improving in some pregnancies and deteriorating in others. It is therefore impossible to predict the likely course of ulcerative colitis in any given patient who becomes pregnant for the second or third time.

The effect of medical treatment for ulcerative colitis on the course and outcome of pregnancy

The two principal agents used in the treatment of ulcerative colitis are sulphasalazine and corticosteroids. Corticosteroids are mainly employed in the treatment of attacks of the disease, while sulphasalazine is most useful as a maintenance therapy to reduce the risk of relapse.

Both of the above drugs have potential hazards which might be of significance in relation to pregnancy. In laboratory animals, corticosteroids may cause resorption of the embryo or congenital abnormalities, particularly fusion failures such as cleft palate (Fraser and Fainstat, 1951; de Costa and Abelman, 1952). An extensive survey of 260 pregnancies during which the mother received cortisone or its analogues suggested that the risk to the human fetus was small (Bongiovanni and McPadden, 1960). However, Warrell and Taylor (1968) took an opposing view. When 34 pregnancies in women receiving prednisolone were compared with the same number of pregnancies in women not receiving steroids but with similar general diseases, the incidence of stillbirth, fetal distress and placental insufficiency was very much higher in the first group. Impaired placental function was suggested to be the cause of the increased fetal risk in the steroid—treated patients.

Sulphasalazine has never been shown to have teratogenic effects in man. However, both the intact drug and its sulphapyridine moiety cross the placenta, and the sulphapyridine may compete with unconjugated bilirubin in the fetal circulation for albumin binding sites (Hensleigh and Kauffman, 1977). Sulphapyridine is also excreted in breast milk, and absorption by the breast-fed child might similarly increase the risk of kernicterus in babies born to mothers receiving sulphasalazine (Järnerot and Into-Malmberg, 1979; Azad Khan and Truelove, 1979). Because of the possible hazards of pathological jaundice in the infant, it has been suggested that sulphasalazine should not be given to women near to parturition.

In Oxford, our current practice is to treat patients with ulcerative colitis who happen to be pregnant in just the same way as we would manage any other patient with the disease. Although the data from our recent survey were not collected in the course of a controlled therapeutic trial, certain comments about the effects of medical therapy can be made.

During the 124 pregnancies which began when the ulcerative colitis was in remission, 45 patients took sulphasalazine treatment throughout pregnancy and 17 of them relapsed (38%), while 76 did not take the drug at all and 18 of them (24%) had recurrences of the disease during pregnancy or the puerperium. The difference is not statistically significant, and the better course in the second group may be attributable in part to the fact that many of these women had been symptom-free for long periods without treatment before they became pregnant. However, we have certainly not identified any dramatic relapse-preventing benefit in the group of patients who continued with their maintenance treatment after conception. On the other hand, sulphasalazine therapy did not have any obvious harmful effect on the outcome of pregnancy. There was no increase in the incidence of congenital malformations in babies born to mothers taking the drug. Pathological jaundice (defined as jaundice requiring special medical treatment) was only slightly more common in infants born to mothers taking sulphasalazine; only one baby required exchange transfusion, and its mother was on no maintenance therapy.

Patients with active ulcerative colitis during pregnancy received a variety of combinations of therapy. Fig. 14.1 shows that the more extensive the treatment required by the mother, the less likely it was

C. P. Willoughby

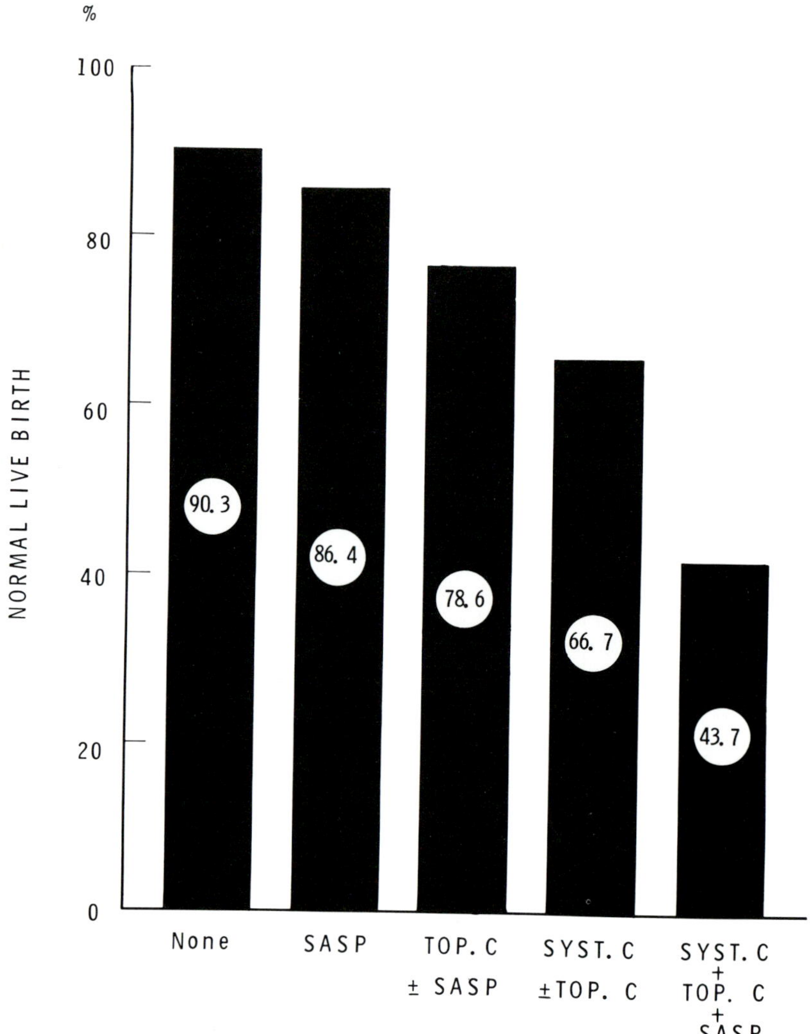

Fig. 14.1. *The proportion of pregnancies resulting in normal live births in relation to the medical treatment received by the mother during the course of pregnancy.*

that the pregnancy would proceed to a normal outcome. Patients who received systemic and topical steroids in addition to sulphasalazine had a particularly unfavourable course, less than half of them producing a normal live baby. Detailed analysis of the results suggests that this poor outlook was probably related to the severity of the ulcerative colitis rather than to the effects of any of the therapeutic agents used. In the whole group, one congenitally abnormal baby (with cerebral palsy) was born prematurely to a steroid-treated mother, while two abnormal children (one of which was also premature) were born to mothers who did not receive corticosteroids. Low birth weight, as an index of placental function, was no commoner in the babies of steroid-treated (18·9%) than of non-steroid-treated patients (18·3%), although the only two stillbirths in the series were produced by steroid-treated mothers. An abnormal degree of neonatal jaundice was no more frequent in the babies of mothers who had taken sulphasalazine throughout pregnancy than in those of women who had not done so.

Pregnancy and surgical treatment of ulcerative colitis

Surgery at the time of pregnancy

In previous surveys, colectomy during or immediately after pregnancy has usually been associated with a bad prognosis for both mother and child. For example, in a series of nine patients reported by McEwan (1972), there were only five normal births. One pregnancy was terminated, two aborted spontaneously and there was one stillbirth. Three of the women died, two during pregnancy and one in the puerperium.

Only two of the patients in our own series were brought to surgery in close temporal relation to a pregnancy. One woman had a therapeutic abortion in an attempt to halt a severe attack of ulcerative colitis, but she continued to deteriorate and was brought to emergency panproctocolectomy, after which she made an uneventful recovery. The other patient had a severe relapse of colitis shortly before delivery; after giving birth to a normal baby, she was transferred to our hospital and was treated by panproctocolectomy, from which she recovered without complications.

Pregnancy after colectomy and ileostomy

Women who have had ulcerative colitis and who have been treated by colectomy and ileostomy have a favourable prognosis as far as pregnancy is concerned. In the past 20 years, five of our patients have had a total of seven pregnancies after proctocolectomy and ileostomy. These pregnancies have not been included in the series discussed above, but a summary of their outcome is presented in Table 14.5, compared with data from previous surveys. As in previous publications, normal live births were the general rule. Minor dysfunction of the stoma occurred late in pregnancy in two patients. Vaginal delivery has been achieved in the majority of cases previously reported, but in our small series three Caesarean sections were performed in two of the women for obstetrical reasons, and normal vaginal delivery occurred in only two pregnancies.

Conclusions

1. The fertility of women with ulcerative colitis seems to be normal.
2. In general, ulcerative colitis has no adverse effect on the outcome of pregnancy. However, patients whose colitis is active at the start of pregnancy have a slightly less favourable prognosis, as far as the result of the pregnancy is concerned, than women whose disease is in remission at the time of conception.
3. If ulcerative colitis is quiescent at the start of pregnancy, there is a good chance that remission will be maintained. If the disease is active at the beginning of pregnancy, 60–70% of patients continue to have symptoms throughout pregnancy and the puerperium. Recurrence or exacerbation of the colitis is particularly likely in the first trimester.
4. As a consequence of the above findings, it seems advisable for patients to achieve a stable remission of their disease before embarking on a pregnancy.
5. Patients who develop ulcerative colitis during pregnancy or the puerperium have a more favourable prognosis than was previously described, and the disease is usually controlled by standard medical treatment.
6. Although the drugs used to treat ulcerative colitis have theoretical hazards when used in pregnancy, these seem to be of little significance in clinical practice. Adverse effects on the outcome of pregnancy are

Table 14.5. *Outcome of pregnancy after colectomy and ileostomy*

Series	Number of pregnancies	Live births	Spontaneous abortion	Therapeutic abortion	Vaginal delivery	Caesarean section	Stomal problems
Banks *et al.* (1957)	9	6	2	1	6	0	1 (unspecified)
Scudamore *et al.* (1957)	7	6	1	0	6	0	1 ileal prolapse 2 intestinal obstruction
de Dombal *et al.* (1965)	6	6	0	0	5	1	0
Roy *et al.* (1970)	35	30	5	0	26	4	1 intestinal obstruction
McEwan (1972)	12	12	0	0	9	3	2 stretching of stoma <u>2</u> intestinal obstruction
	—	—	—	—	—	—	(1 maternal death)
Total	69	60 (87%)	8 (12%)	1	52	8	9 (13%)
Oxford series (1980)	7	5 (71%)	2 (29%)	0	2	3	2 (minor leakage around appliance)

probably more closely related to the severity of the colitis than to the agents used in its treatment.

7. Patients who have had ulcerative colitis and who have been treated by colectomy and ileostomy have a good chance of a normal outcome to any subsequent pregnancies. Significant ileostomy problems during pregnancy are relatively uncommon.

References

Abramson D., Jankelson I.R. and Milner L.R. (1951) *Amer. J. Obst. Gynec.* **61**, 121.

Azad Khan A.K. and Truelove S.C. (1979) *Brit. med. J.* ii, 1553.

Banks B.M., Korelitz B.I. and Zetzel L. (1957) *Gastroenterology,* **32**, 983.

Bongiovanni A.M. and McPadden A.J. (1960) *Fertil. Steril.* **11**, 181.

Crohn B.B., Yarnis H., Crohn E.B., Walter R.I. and Gabrilove L.J. (1956) *Gastro-enterology,* **30**, 391.

de Costa E.J. and Abelman M.A. (1952) *Amer. J. Obst. Gynec.* **64**, 746.

de Dombal F.T., Watts J.M., Watkinson G. and Goligher J.C. (1965) *Lancet,* ii, 599.

Donald I. (1974) *Practical Obstetrical Problems,* 4th ed. Lloyd-Luke, London.

Fraser F.C. and Fainstat T.D. (1951) *Pediatrics,* **8**, 527.

Gossage A.M. and Price F.W. (1909) *Proc. roy. Soc. Med.* **2**, (Medical Section), 151.

Harrison R.F. (1977). In: *Contemporary Obstetrics and Gynecology* ed. Chamberlain G.V.P. Northwood Publications, London, p. 308.

Hensleigh P.A. and Kauffman R.E. (1977) *Amer. J. Obst. Gynec.* **127**, 443.

Järnerot G. and Into-Malmberg M.B. (1979) *Scand. J. Gastroenterol.* **14**, 869.

Kleckner M.S., Bargen J.A. and Banner E.A. (1951) *Amer. J. Obst. Gynec.* **62**, 1234.

MacDougall I. (1956) *Lancet,* ii, 641.

McEwan H.P. (1972) *Proc. roy. Soc. Med.* **65**, 279.

Roy P.H., Sauer W.G., Beahrs O.H. and Farrow G.M. (1970) *Amer. J. Surg.* **119**, 77.

Scudamore H.H., Rogers A.G., Bargen J.A. and Banner E.A. (1957) *Gastro-enterology,* **32**, 295.

Stevenson A.C., Dudgeon M.Y. and McClure H.I. (1959) *Ann. hum. Genet.* **23**, 395.

Warrell D.W. and Taylor R. (1968) *Lancet,* i, 117.

Webb M.J. and Sedlack R.E. (1974) *Med. Clin. N. Amer.* **58**, 823.

Willoughby C.P. and Truelove S.C. (1980) *Gut,* **21**, 469.

Zetzel L. (1954) *New Engl. J. Med.* **251**, 610.

Chapter 15
Prevention of cancer

S. C. TRUELOVE

It is well established that patients with chronic ulcerative colitis are unduly prone to suffer from cancer of the large bowel. As a result, one of the most important objectives in the management of patients with ulcerative colitis is to prevent, as far as possible, the occurrence of this dangerous complication. Before proceeding to a discussion of how this objective may be achieved, it is helpful to consider some of the special features of cancer complicating ulcerative colitis, including its time of occurrence.

Special features

1. The cancer frequently occurs in patients who are comparatively young.
2. The malignant growths are frequently multiple.
3. The distribution of the growths is different from that observed in the general population because they are liable to occur in any part of the large bowel with roughly equal frequency whereas in the general population about 75% occur in the rectum or lower sigmoid colon.

Time of occurrence and magnitude of risk

During the first few years after the onset of ulcerative colitis, the risk of developing cancer is small. Thereafter the risk becomes appreciable and especially after the colitis has been present for more than ten years. In order to assess the risk with some precision, it is necessary to follow a large group of patients from the time of their first attack and then to use actuarial methods to handle the data for reasons which have been

cogently expressed by Devroede and Taylor (1976). Figure 15.1 shows
the results obtained in an Oxford survey in which both these conditions
were met and, in addition, the follow-up was complete for all the
patients. It will be seen that very few cases of cancer of the large bowel
occurred during the first seven years of follow-up, but that thereafter
there was a continued liability to develop this complication. This
survey covered the period 1938–1962 when radical surgery was used
much less than it is today for the treatment of ulcerative colitis and the
survey therefore gives a fairly good picture of the cancer risk inherent
in chronic ulcerative colitis and which we nowadays seek to minimize.

Another study which gives an idea of the magnitude of the cancer
risk in ulcerative colitis is that of Nefzger and Acheson (1963). This
was a study of the mortality and cancer risk in 525 men admitted to
U.S. Army hospitals in 1944 compared with matched controls drawn
from the U.S. Army. The period of follow-up was 17 years, and at the
end of this time the deaths in the ulcerative colitis group were double
those in the control group. About 50% of the excess mortality in the
subjects with ulcerative colitis was attributable to cancer of the large
bowel, which occurred during the later years of the follow-up period.

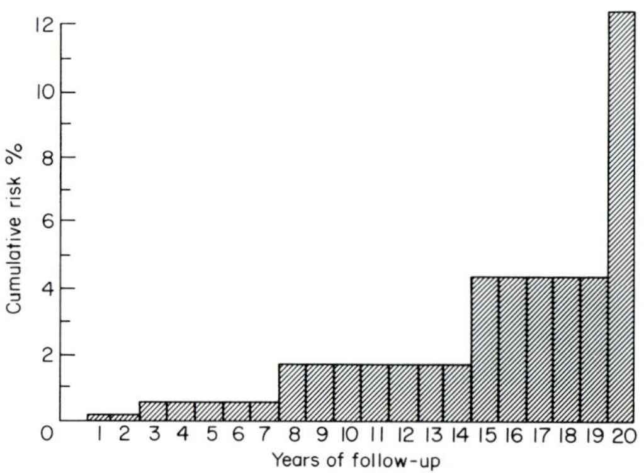

Fig. 15.1. *Cumulative percentage risk of developing cancer of the large bowel
in patients with ulcerative colitis, based on the findings in 250 patients seen
in their first attack of ulcerative colitis and then followed up. Note that the
number of patients followed for 20 years or more was small so little attention
should be paid to the sharp increase at 20 years as this estimate of the risk
may be falsely high. (From Edwards and Truelove, 1964).*

Methods of prevention

There are two main approaches to the problem of how to prevent cancer of the large bowel in patients with ulcerative colitis:

1. The clinical approach relies upon recognising a sub-group of ulcerative colitis patients who are at special risk of developing cancer and then employing prophylactic proctocolectomy in order to eliminate this risk.
2. The histological approach relies upon the recognition of epithelial dysplasia in mucosal biopsy specimens as an indication that the patient is at special risk of developing cancer, or may have already done so.

These two approaches will now be discussed in some detail:

1. The clinical approach

Although patients with ulcerative colitis have an increased liability to develop cancer of the large bowel, this risk does not apply equally to all patients with ulcerative colitis. It is possible to define certain features which mean that patients who possess them are at considerable risk. In a study of the course and prognosis of ulcerative colitis that we made at Oxford (Edwards and Truelove, 1964), the following features emerged as indicating a special risk of cancer when the ulcerative colitis had been present for more than ten years:

1. A clinically severe first attack of the disease (which usually implies widespread damage to the colonic mucosa).

2. Universal or very extensive involvement of the colon as judged radiologically.

3. Chronic continuous symptoms from the colitis as opposed to the more usual type of intermittent course in which there are attacks of colitis with periods of complete freedom from symptoms in between the attacks. The patients with chronic continuous symptoms had five times the risk of developing cancer as had those with intermittent symptoms.

4. Onset of the ulcerative colitis in childhood or adolescence. Such patients frequently have universal colitis but there seems to be a special liability for them to develop cancer as a late complication even allowing for this. The formidable risk of cancer in such patients has been well documented by Devroede *et al.* (1971). (See also Chapter 13.)

As a result of these findings, my own policy since 1965 has been to recommend a prophylactic proctocolectomy in patients with two or more of the above features when the ulcerative colitis has been present for more than ten years, even if the colitis had become quiescent. In the event, such a recommendation is necessary in only a small number of patients purely for the purpose of preventing cancer. The four clinical features which are associated with a high risk of cancer are also features which imply that the ulcerative colitis is likely to run a severe course. The result is that many of the patients with a combination of two or more of these features have already been treated by proctocolectomy before the ulcerative colitis has been in existence for more than ten years. During the past 12 years, only 13 of my patients have been treated by proctocolectomy for the sole reason that the operation was to eliminate the risk of cancer. In any event, the policy has been fairly successful in reducing the cancer risk to tolerable proportions. During the past seven years, with our ulcerative colitis clinic averaging around 750 regular attenders, there have been only four cases of cancer of the large bowel, all of which have been small and apparently cured by proctocolectomy. One of these was recognized by the histological approach which is dealt with later. (I have excluded from these considerations two patients referred to me from other hospitals who had already developed a cancer of the large bowel by the time of referral.)

The converse of the finding that certain factors are associated with a specially high cancer risk in ulcerative colitis is that the absence of any of these factors in a patient means that he is not at any undue risk of developing a cancer of the large bowel. In other words, when a patient develops ulcerative colitis in adult life, provided that the disease is distal and that the attacks of colitis are intermittent, the risk of his developing a cancer is too small to justify a prophylactic proctocolectomy.

A basically similar approach to the one already covered has also been employed by Bonnevie *et al.* (1974) and they had no case of cancer developing in 332 patients with ulcerative colitis whom they dealt with between 1964 and 1971. Likewise, Kristensen *et al.* (1977) used radical surgery freely in the treatment of 296 patients during the period 1964–74. Four of their patients had cancer of the colon but in three of these the tumour was already present by the time the patient was referred to their hospital.

It therefore appears that prophylactic proctocolectomy carried out on a selected sample of ulcerative colitis patients can reduce the cancer risk to a low level, albeit at the price of a large operation and life with a permanent ileostomy thereafter.

2. The histological approach

This approach to the prevention of cancer in ulcerative colitis had its origins in the observations of Morson and Pang (1967). They made a detailed study of colectomy specimens from patients with ulcerative colitis complicated by cancer of the large bowel and they found that such specimens frequently showed a widespread epithelial dysplasia. This dysplasia, which is sometimes known as the 'Morson lesion', was considered by them to be a precancerous condition. They therefore deduced that regular rectal biopsy would detect such a change and would assist in the early detection of cancer or indicate the need for prophylactic colectomy.

During the past decade, the development of colonoscopy has greatly enlarged the scope of this approach as it means that multiple biopsy specimens can be obtained from all areas of the large bowel, with a correspondingly greater chance of finding evidence of dysplasia or frank carcinoma.

Lennard-Jones *et al.* (1974) reported on the progress of 171 patients with extensive or universal colitis followed in their outpatient department during the period 1966–1973. Three of the patients developed cancer of the large bowel and they all showed dysplastic changes on rectal biopsy. Eleven other patients showed dysplasia in their rectal biopsy specimens and four of them were treated by colectomy but no cancer was found. A subsequent report from the same group dealt with 229 patients observed for ten years; seven of them who consistently showed severe dysplasia in their rectal or colonic biopsy specimens were treated by colectomy and cancer was found in four of them; in all four, the cancer was confined to the bowel wall (Duke's A), suggesting the possibility of a good prognosis (Lennard–Jones *et al.*, 1977). Other workers have also suggested that the finding of widespread dysplasia indicates a strong possibility that a cancer has already developed.

As a result, it has been suggested that colonoscopy with multiple biopsy should be performed every two years in patients with universal or extensive colitis and more frequently if there are any suspicious findings (Lennard–Jones *et al.*, 1977). This is a formidable programme and it remains to be seen whether the results justify the means.

In any event, it can be seen that the histological approach is far from perfect. Rectal biopsy may have shown dysplasia but colectomy may reveal no cancer. Conversely, if colonoscopy with biopsy is performed every two years, there must be the possibility that a cancer may develop during the intervals.

In addition, the recognition of dysplasia calls for histopathologists with good experience of ulcerative colitis. The possibility of error arises because the colonic epithelium frequently shows dysplastic features in the presence of active inflammation, only to revert to normal when the inflammation subsides. For the dysplasia to be a significant indicator of a precancerous state, it appears that it must be present when the colitis is in a quiescent phase.

Combining the two approaches

The two methods that I have described for minimising the cancer risk in ulcerative colitis should not be looked upon as mutually exclusive. In principle, the clinical approach could be used to define the sub-population of ulcerative colitis patients who are at special risk of developing a cancer, and then, instead of recommending them to be treated by prophylactic colectomy, it would be possible to monitor them by regular colonoscopic multiple biopsy and to proceed to proctocolectomy only if there were evidence of definite dysplasia. The ideal would be to set up long-term studies in which the two main methods would be compared and also the type of combined approach now suggested. The amount of work involved in such comparative studies would be great but without such studies it is difficult to see how we shall ever arrive at the most effective method for dealing with the problem of how to combat the cancer risk in chronic ulcerative colitis.

An unknown factor

One of the great difficulties in assessing the best approach to the cancer risk in ulcerative colitis arises from the fact that the cancer seldom occurs before the ulcerative colitis has been in existence for more than ten years. The result is that it will be necessary to wait for many years before it is possible to see whether modern medical therapy has diminished the cancer risk in this disease. As most attacks of ulcerative colitis are mild and can be cut short by cortico-steroid therapy if this is promptly instituted, and as recurrences are sharply reduced in number by maintenance treatment with sulphasala-zine (Misiewicz *et al.*, 1965; Dissanayake & Truelove, 1973), there is a distinct possibility that patients developing ulcerative colitis today have a lower chance of developing cancer as a late complication than did patients who first developed the disease more than a decade ago. It is certainly my own experience that the risk of cancer in patients under regular supervision and treatment in an ulcerative colitis clinic nowadays appears to be quite small, but only laborious follow-up studies with actuarial analysis of the data will enable this impression to be put to the test.

Conclusions

One of the late complications of ulcerative colitis is cancer of the large bowel. The cancer frequently affects comparatively young patients, is sometimes multiple, and occurs with roughly equal frequency in all parts of the large bowel. There are two main methods of reducing the cancer risk. The clinical approach relies upon defining the factors associated with a specially high risk of cancer and employing prophy-lactic proctocolectomy in selected patients with two or more bad-risk factors. The histological approach relies upon the finding of epithelial dysplasia in rectal or colonic biopsy specimens to indicate that a cancer has already developed or, even if not, that prophylactic colectomy is justifiable. Neither method is perfect and further studies are required to define which is the better course to follow, or whether some combi-nation of the two is to be preferred.

ACKNOWLEDGEMENT

Figure 15.1 is reproduced by permission of the Editor of *Gut*.

References

Bonnevie O., Binder V., Anthonisen P. *et al.* (1974) *Scand. J. Gastroenterol.* **9**, 81.
Devroede G. and Taylor W.F. (1976) *Gastroenterology,* **71**, 505.
Devroede G., Taylor W.F., Sauer W.G., *et al.* (1971) *New Engl. J. Med.* **285**, 17.
Dissanayake A.S. and Truelove S.C. (1973) *Gut,* **14**, 923.

Edwards F.C. and Truelove S.C. (1964) *Gut,* **5**, 15.

Kristensen M., Koudahl G. and Jarnum S. (1977) *Ugeskr. Laeg.* **139**, 2377.

Lennard—Jones J.E., Misiewicz J.J., Parrish J.A., Ritchie J.K. *et al.* (1974) *Lancet,* i, 1065.

Lennard—Jones J.E., Morson B.C., Ritchie J.K. *et al.* (1977) *Gastroenterology,* **73**, 1280.

Misiewicz J.J., Lennard-Jones J.E., Connell A.M. *et al.* (1965) *Lancet,* **i**, 185.

Morson B.C. and Pang L.S.C. (1967) *Gut,* **8**, 423.

Nefzger M.D. and Acheson E.D. (1963) *Gut,* **4**, 183

Chapter 16
Proctocolectomy

EMANOEL C. G. LEE

Although the majority of patients with ulcerative colitis can be looked after successfully for life by medical treatment alone, a proportion still come to operation. Surgery may be required during an attack when the severity of the colitis makes it essential for the colon to be removed to save the patient's life. An operation may be undertaken electively in patients suffering from severe troublesome attacks or from continuous incapacitating symptoms. Less commonly, the indication for surgical treatment may be as a prophylactic measure in patients who are considered to be at high risk of developing cancer. It is our opinion that, for all these purposes, the operation of proctocolectomy as a single-stage procedure has stood the test of time as the technique of choice in the majority of patients (Lee and Truelove, 1980).

Operations during an acute attack of colitis

A severe attack of colitis is still a dangerous condition which requires the prompt attention of a trained gastroenterological team. Preferably the team should consist of surgeons and physicians with specialised experience and who are accustomed to working closely together. The prognosis of a severe attack has improved since the early 1950's when, even in the best units, nearly 30% of such patients died from the attack while in hospital. The improvement can be attributed partly to the use of corticosteroids and partly to the adoption of early surgery for patients who do not respond rapidly to medical treatment.

The current technique of medical treatment has evolved gradually. At first, oral corticosteroids were used and were often continued for quite long periods; now we use a short intensive regimen of prednisolone given intravenously. It is our practice to maintain the intravenous regimen for five days in combination with careful control of fluid, electrolytes and haemoglobin. We then administer prednisolone by the oral route in fairly large doses before tailing it off after about a month. The results of the technique over the past ten years have been reviewed in two studies (Truelove and Jewell, 1974; Truelove *et al.*, 1978). Two-thirds to three-quarters·of the patients respond promptly and are in complete clinical remission by the end of five days. Some patients show no improvement or become worse on the regimen and it is our policy to carry out emergency surgery in such patients. Patients requiring emergency surgery can be divided into three groups:

1. Patients who are admitted with a perforation of the colon are treated by an emergency proctocolectomy on the day of admission. Likewise, some patients admitted with acute dilatation of the colon are treated by immediate proctocolectomy, if the degree of dilatation is severe.

2. Patients who develop acute dilatation or perforation while on the five day regimen have emergency surgery.

3. Patients who respond well to the five day regimen, but who suffer from a recrudescence of the attack when the intravenous regimen is discontinued, are usually treated by urgent surgery.

Since the introduction of the five day regimen in Oxford, no patient has died while on the medical treatment and the operative mortality has been just over 2%. The introduction of early surgery as pioneered by Goligher and his colleagues at Leeds resulted in a drop in the surgical mortality from over 20% in the decade before 1963 to about 7% (Goligher *et al.*, 1970). The combined regimen of medical and surgical treatment outlined above has improved the results further.

The choice of operative technique
during an acute attack

Although in the past surgeons advocated limited surgery for acute dilatation of the colon (such as appendicostomy, diversionary ileostomy or, more recently, the multiple 'blow-hole' colostomies advocated by Turnbull), we have found that a more radical operation has yielded better results. Since 1970, we have employed a single-stage proctocolectomy using the technique of perimuscular dissection of the rectum during the operation even when it is being carried out as an emergency. The rectum has been retained in only a small number of patients. In some of these, the rectum was entirely normal and it was suspected that the patient might be suffering from Crohn's disease rather than ulcerative colitis. In a few patients with undoubted ulcerative colitis, there was an unusual degree of relative sparing of the rectum. Finally, there was an occasional patient in whom the rectum was retained because a full proctocolectomy seemed to carry too high a risk; for example, a patient with haemophilia and severe acute colitis was treated initially by a subtotal colectomy and the rectum was removed later as a separate operation.

We have carried out the operation of single-stage proctocolectomy as an emergency in 48 patients with one death. These results should be compared with previous reports in which the mortality varied between 40% (Ritchie, 1971) and 25% for the operation of subtotal colectomy with an ileostomy, the distal colon being retained as a mucous fistula (Koudahl and Kristensen, 1976). In the past, it was our experience that a considerable proportion of the morbidity which occurred after a subtotal colectomy was due to intraperitoneal sepsis, wound sepsis or septicaemia. Many of these infective complications could be traced directly to sepsis around the retained rectum. At the time, we had already developed the technique of perimuscular dissection of the rectum for elective proctocolectomy and this had virtually eliminated the major postoperative problem of impotence (Lee and Dowling, 1972). We were thus encouraged to remove the rectum by the same technique in the emergency cases as well. Other surgeons, such as Walker (1969), Scott *et al.* (1970) and Jones *et al.* (1977), have also reported a reduction in the mortality after single-stage proctocolectomy was introduced as the emergency procedure.

However the technique is not a simple one, and it is not advocated as the emergency operation of choice for an inexperienced surgeon faced with a severely ill patient in a hospital in which there are few resources for postoperative management. Perhaps it is for this situation that Turnbull *et al.* (1971) advocated 'blow-hole' colostomies to relieve distension and an ileostomy to divert faecal contents in patients with severe dilatation of the colon. It is suggested that excisional surgery carries a major risk of perforation of the colon when the bowel is being handled, with the result that the peritoneum may be flooded with faeces. It has been our experience that, if a careful technique of dissection is employed, such leakage can usually be prevented even though the patient has free perforations or multiple sealed perforations.

Proctocolectomy for patients with chronic disease

The majority of patients who come to surgery for the treatment of
ulcerative colitis do so as elective cases because of repeated troublesome
exacerbations of colitis or because the symptoms are continuous in
spite of the most careful medical treatment. In addition, a small group
of patients require the operation because of the development of a complication such as a stricture, carcinoma or fistula. Other complications,
particularly the remote or systemic ones, such as pyodermia gangreno-
sum, arthritis and eye changes, are not now considered to be indications
for surgery since they usually respond speedily to corticosteroid therapy.
Ankylosing spondylitis, on the other hand, does not usually respond to
medical or surgical treatment and is therefore not a factor in influencing
a decision for or against surgery.

Elective surgery should be performed after careful preparation of the
patient, which involves both physical and psychological aspects. The
patient should, of course, not be anaemic and should be maintained in
the best possible state of nutrition. If the patient has suffered weight-
loss or malnutrition, a pre-operative period of intensive intravenous
feeding is advisable. Psychological preparation of the patient to deal
with a permanent ileostomy is perhaps the most important aspect of
pre-operative management (Chapter 18).

The choice of operation as an elective procedure

Although many surgeons prefer to retain the rectum for re-anastomosis
after a subtotal colectomy, during which an ileostomy and mucous
fistula is fashioned, or a single-stage ileo-rectal anastomosis is undertaken, our preference in the majority of cases is for a single-stage
proctocolectomy combined with a Brooke-type eversion ileostomy.
This has the advantage that the whole of the diseased organ is removed
as a primary procedure, thus avoiding a second operation, which is
often necessary when the rectum is retained. Mortality is similar for
both types of procedure, as judged from the literature, being of the
order of 3% in specialised centres. Although there are some complications associated with an ileostomy, most of these occur during the
first 18 months post-operatively. Subsequently, the majority of patients
do well and the long-term results are excellent, with survival approaching
that of the general population (Ritchie, 1971).

There are two main points which can be made against proctocolec-tomy:

1. Autonomic nerves in the pelvis may be damaged during dissection and a patient may therefore end up with total bladder dysfunction as well as impotence (in the male) or loss of orgasm (in the female). These sequelae were distinct possibilities when surgeons carried out wide dissections in the pelvis using the same technique that was employed during a synchronous abdomino-perineal excision of the rectum for a carcinoma. A number of technical improvements were introduced in the sixties, such as a low ligation of the inferior mesenteric vessels, a careful dissection of the lateral posterior ligaments surrounding the rectum, the preservation of the parasympathetic nerves in the pelvis and the retention of the levator muscles. These techniques reduced the post-operative complications, but permanent impotence was still recorded in quite a high proportion of young men.

Both sympathetic and parasympathetic nervous systems are required for completely normal functioning of the bladder and sex organs. In addition, a normal arrangement of the layers of the pelvis is necessary for bladder function and to prevent problems during intercourse in women after proctocolectomy.

In 1970, we introduced the technique of dissecting the rectum in the perimuscular plane from above and in the intermuscular plane from below (Lee and Dowling, 1972). This has virtually eliminated the bladder and sexual dysfunction which often followed proctectomy. In addition, it is possible to close all layers of the pelvis, including the peritoneum, extra-peritoneal fat, levator muscles, fascia covering the ischiorectal fascia, subcutaneous tissue and skin. We do not now leave a drain through the middle of the perineal wound to drain the pelvis, as this often led to a persistent perineal sinus. At present, we do not drain the pelvis from below, but only drain the deep layers of the pelvis with a suction tube brought out on the left side of the abdomen.

2. The other disadvantage of proctectomy arises from problems associated with the permanent ileostomy. These are now minor, and it is our opinion that, in the past, many of them were due to inadequate pre- and post-operative management of the patient.

Recently, a number of surgeons have been advocating the operation of subtotal colectomy with ileorectal anastomosis in order to avoid a permanent ileostomy. This operation can be carried out in one stage, or an ileostomy can be made with a mucous fistula of the distal sigmoid, and the continuity of the bowel can be restored subsequently. Aylett has recorded exceptionally good results after ileo-rectal anastomosis which he employs almost exclusively in the treatment of patients with ulcerative colitis (Aylett, 1974, 1976). Other surgeons have found the proportion of cases in which the operation can be undertaken to be much less than Aylett advocated, between 6 and 40 per cent of cases having been reported as being suitable for the operation. Our own experience is that about 10% of cases are suitable for an ileo-rectal anastomosis. It has also been our experience that the majority of patients on whom the operation is performed continue to have active inflammation in the rectum post-operatively and some may develop such severe acute attacks of proctitis (which may induce remote complications such as arthropathies and skin disease) that we have been forced to excise the retained rectum, sometimes almost as an emergency. Even when an immediate anastomosis is not carried out, the majority of our patients continue to have inflammation in the defunctioned rectum and many require proctectomy without ever being considered for restorative anastomosis. This is particularly true in the patients who have had a colectomy as an emergency procedure for a severe attack of ulcerative colitis.

The major disadvantage of an ileo-rectal anastomosis is that the rectum has an appreciable chance of becoming the site for a carcinoma. Aylett recorded 12 patients with cancer after 461 operations, but evidence is now accumulating that the rate of carcinoma may be as high as 10%. What is worse is that these tumours may develop suddenly. Many are difficult to diagnose because early symptoms, such as an increased frequency of stools and minor rectal bleeding, may be mistaken by the patient and even by the surgeon as an inflammatory episode and a tumour may spread widely before the rectum can be excised. Because of the high rate of malignancy, even those who strongly advocate ileo-rectal anastomosis have suggested that the operation is most suitable as an interim procedure, particularly in young people, who may thus be able to continue with natural defaecation for several years before the rectum needs to be removed.

In spite of reports of normal post-operative bowel function in the majority of patients after an ileo-rectal anastomosis, it has been our experience that more than half the patients suffer from troublesome diarrhoea. No one has yet tried to assess whether the problems of a permanent ileostomy are greater or less than the problems of diarrhoea after an ileo-rectal anastomosis.

At the present time, although most surgeons and physicians are agreed about the indications for surgery in ulcerative colitis, there is still a considerable difference of opinion about the type of operation which should be used. In Britain, the majority of surgeons carry out a proctocolectomy with a permanent ileostomy, but a significant number consider that an ileo-rectal anastomosis is superior. A categorical opinion as to which is the better operation cannot be given because they have never been compared in a controlled trial and at present the choice of operation to be advocated must rest with the individual surgeon concerned. It is our opinion that proctocolectomy has the major advantage that the patient is cured of the disease and that problems that arise afterwards can be equated with the symptoms following an ileo-rectal anastomosis without the threat hanging over the patient that a cancer may occur at any time.

References

Aylett S.O. (1974) *Arch. Mal. App. dig.* **63**, 585.
Aylett S.O. (1976). In *A Surgical Division*, ed. Clarke T.K. Squibb. London.
Goligher J.C., Hoffman D.C. and de Dombal F.T. (1970) *Brit. med. J.* **iv**, 703.
Jones P.F., Munroe A. and Ewen S.W.B. (1977) *Brit. J. Surg.* **64**, 615.
Koudahl G. and Kristensen M. (1976) *Scand. J. Gastroenterol.* (Suppl), **137**, 117.
Lee E.C.G. and Dowling B.L. (1972) *Brit. J. Surg.* **59**, 29.
Lee E.C.G. and Truelove S.C. (1980) *World J. Surg.* **4**, 195.
Ritchie J.K. (1971) *Gut,* **12**, 528.
Scott H.W., Wimberley J.E., Shull H.J. and Law D.H. IV (1970) *Amer. J. Surg.* **119**, 87.
Truelove S.C. and Jewell D.P. (1974) *Lancet,* i, 1067.
Truelove S.C., Willoughby C.P., Lee E.C.G. and Kettlewell M.G.W. (1978) *Lancet,* ii, 1086.
Turnbull R.B. Jr., Hawk W.A. and Weakley F.L. (1971) *Amer. J. Surg.* **122**, 325.
Walker F.C. (1969) *The Surgical Management of Ulcerative Colitis.* Butterworths, London.

Chapter 17

Life with an ileostomy

AN ILEOSTOMIST

Editorial Comment
The author of this chapter is a scientist who had a distinguished
university career before moving into research with a large pharmaceutical
company, of which he is now a senior executive on the research side.
He is a man of exceptional vitality, both physical and mental. His
account of his own illness illustrates vividly how a person can adapt
completely to life with an ileostomy. We realise, from our own
experience with other patients, that there is a wide range of reaction
among them to the problems presented by a permanent ileostomy, as is
dealt with to some extent in Chapters 18 and 19.

In this chapter, I shall try to give a picture of my situation before and
immediately after my proctocolectomy, and of my ten years' experience
of life with an ileostomy. Perhaps I can crystallize my attitude best by
suggesting that the title of this chapter ought to be 'My ileostomy's life
with me'. Put simply, I can say that the allowances I have had to make
as an ileostomist have been few and minor. My approach has been to
expect the ileostomy to tolerate all my needs and desires, be they
professional, social, gastronomic or sexual. Although I have not previously bothered to dwell on my pre-operative state, I can readily recall
that it was unmitigated hell.

Pre-operative state

At first, following a severe episode of ulcerative colitis in 1962 which
required three weeks medical treatment and hospitalization, intensive
and prolonged steroid therapy allowed me to lead a normal life. I gained
a lot of weight and this gave the impression of improved health. During

the next eight years, apart from occasional attacks of symptoms, I was clearly accommodating to a level of disease and incapacity which steadily and almost imperceptibly worsened.

This was a particularly important period in my career. For some months before my operation in 1969, I unconsciously concentrated all my efforts on my job. Thus, entirely due to my own neglect and refusal to accept my situation, I came to operation in a poor state, with widespread disease in my colon and with a large abscess. Pain had increased during the last pre-operative year. At first this was simply discomfort, but it then developed into attacks of acute abdominal pain as food attempted to squeeze past inflamed areas in a widely diseased colon. Eventually, these attacks of pain became quite disabling. At the same time, I suffered from increasing fatigue, sensitivity to cold and loss of concentration. The result was that I needed to sleep more and more, so that eventually I was either at work or in bed. In effect, I ended up working to survive and surviving only to work.

Far and away the worst feature was the constant feeling of general malaise. This is difficult to describe completely. Food, however delectable to others, produced episodes of nausea and diarrhoea with increasing frequency. Travel was a nightmare. Road journeys needed to be measured in terms of the miles between toilet facilities owing to the frequency of diarrhoea. Travel by air, especially to foreign countries, presented almost insurmountable problems, although I somehow managed to devise solutions.

Immediate post-operative experience

Such was the state into which I had fallen, entirely due to my self-neglect and my determination to continue work at all costs, that, when I was told that immediate surgery was essential, my initial shock rapidly evaporated at the prospect of relief from my illness. I could not have been a more willing subject, even though, having watched the X-ray monitor, I was generally aware of the extent and severity of the disease. The nature of the operative procedure was carefully explained to me and, although I could imagine the consequences, I just wanted to get on with it without delay. Despite my willingness to submit to surgery, I could not have expected the supreme feeling of well-being that I experienced 48 hours after surgery. Steroids obviously helped, as well as post-operative analgesia, but somehow there was also an indescribable feeling of release from the general malaise.

My recovery was rapid. I was out of bed on day two and walking round the ward on day three. I began to eat semi-solids on day four and made more extensive perambulations. I had an incredible sense of well-being, especially mental well-being, such as I had not previously experienced. I dictated papers that I was due to present at a scientific meeting to be held six weeks later. Taste and appetite returned immediately. Steady progress was made under excellent nursing care. Ileostomy function was excellent, the effluent beginning to solidify within a few days. The management of the ileostomy was readily learned and I even taught on it to student nurses on day nine. Walking the hospital corridor and escaping temporarily for tea with my wife and children in the beautiful little town of Broadway helped in my rapid recovery. I was discharged from the ward on day ten just after an illicit but superb celebration with champagne and caviar in a side ward with all the medical and nursing staff who were able to participate. I myself could taste and thoroughly enjoy both of these delicacies.

Convalescence at home

Such was the excellent state of my psyche following my release from a living hell that I wanted to get back to work as soon as possible. I immediately drove my car but this tore the stitches out of my perineal wound and I therefore had to forego this activity for some weeks. Instead, I monitored my improving strength by riding my daughter's bicycle each day over a standard route of about 4 kilometres and recording times which demonstrated steady improvement. After three weeks, I was back at work, sleeping normally and luxuriating in eating and being alive.

Sexual function took longer to return. Erection was painful for some while and became normal only after six months or so. The pain early on made me wonder if my surgeon had found the need for an accessory restraining device on the operating table!

Subsequent recovery

Ileostomy function became efficient, regular and predictable. The effluent was rarely excessively fluid and nowadays never is unless I drink cheap red wine. Alcohol usually reduces rather than increases the viscosity of the effluent, although I am told that this is unusual. Management of the ileostomy was no problem, thanks to the invaluable help from a stoma therapist who supplied advice and equipment.

Long-term experience

Accidents can happen with an ileostomy and they often did in the early days. Usually they arose from neglect or from an over-enthusiastic approach to energetic physical activities. Even these incidents have diminished, so much so that it must be several years since I last experienced one. The equipment is so good that intervals between changes of 10–14 days are routine for me. The procedure takes me only a few minutes.

I have never let the ileostomy prevent me from engaging in any kind of physical activity. I am accustomed to drive long distances at a stretch. For some years I took part in rallies which lasted all night and even today I am capable of driving up to 800 miles in a single day. While my job calls for little physical activity, most of my leisure is taken up with purposeful activity rather than sports or games. One of my great hobbies is motor engineering and I enjoy rebuilding motor cars, in addition to normal servicing and repairs.

Eating is an absolute joy. Before my operation, my diet had always been severely restricted both from choice and lack of interest. Now there is virtually nothing that I do not eat and any selection is conscious and not from necessity. Only cheap red wine seems to increase peristalsis and then in only a transient manner. Unfortunately, I love cheap red wine!

Travel abroad is a delight. Gut infections which lay others low cause me only minor disturbance and are of short duration. They seem to occur less and less. The sheer convenience of an ileostomy in circumstances of restricted access to bathroom facilities has to be experienced to be appreciated. I have no wish to return to the 'normal' procedures.

The effects on sexual relationships are interesting. After a slow start, I decided (being a scientist) that in this, as in all things, single observations are unreliable. On the basis of a small and uncontrolled study, I am pleased to report that, all other things being equal, an ileostomy makes no significant difference to the joy and delight of prolonged and frequent lovemaking. If mechanical problems arise they can readily be solved.

Are there any disadvantages? Well, maybe I have been lucky, but I have found none. I can imagine people living in cramped home circumstances, or those having other physical or mental problems, for whom an ileostomy would be a burden. For me, the joy of leading a far more normal and productive life than I experienced even before I became ill is overriding. I cannot sufficiently express my gratitude to all those clever, efficient and caring people who have put me where I am today.

Chapter 18
Role of the stoma therapist

PENNY KANE

It is only in recent years that the Department of Health has recognised the need for a specialist nurse, trained in stoma therapy, to work within the National Health Service. Previously the care of ostomists, in hospital, was undertaken by overworked staff who often had little or no experience of stoma care. In addition, on returning home, many ostomists had little or no help in dealing with any difficulties encountered with their stoma.

In many parts of this country, the stoma therapist has responsibility for stoma care in a whole district, which usually includes two or more hospitals as well as the local community. In every case the stoma therapist should ensure that the patients whom she has looked after in hospital have good care on returning home.

Main aim

The stoma therapist is appointed with the sole function of assisting ostomists and their families. She works as part of a team of doctors, nurses, social workers and dietitians. The main aim is to train the patient in self care so that he is able to continue with his normal job, carry on with his family responsibilities and engage in his normal social activities. This is particularly important with ileostomists as many of them are young and have most of their lives before them. Various aspects of stoma therapy will be discussed in this chapter.

Preoperative care

Wherever possible the patient should be seen before the operation. Pre-operative counselling may play an important part in helping the patient adapt rapidly to life with a stoma. At the first interview, assessment should be made of the patient's psychological make-up, physical state and socio-economic background. All these factors are important in determining the way in which a patient is likely to adapt to life with a stoma.

Explanation of the operation using simple terms and diagrams, and discussion of the consequent effect on the patient's future life, may do much to allay his fears and anxieties. Many patients fear that having a stoma will render them crippled and useless, so that they will become a burden on their families. Few people understand the long and often complicated terms that we so often use when describing anatomy and physiology. The stoma therapist must be an attentive and perceptive listener, so that she can recognise any unnecessary fears and anxieties. It is important that the information given to the patient should be the same from all sources, otherwise he becomes confused and fearful.

Usually it is helpful to show the patient an ileostomy appliance that is commonly recommended by the stoma therapist and to discuss how it is obtained, stored and disposed of. Other topics which should be discussed are employment, diet, clothing, social activities and sexual life. It is also reassuring to the patient if he is told what his treatment will be during the first few postoperative days. Nasogastric tubes, catheters, drainage tubes and intravenous infusions are frightening unless they are known to be part of the normal treatment.

Some patients are eager for knowledge but others are not. Invariably, we find that it is very helpful for the patient if a meeting is arranged with an ileostomist of similar age, sex and social background. The two should be given the opportunity for a long discussion under conditions of privacy.

The stoma site should be marked to ensure the best position. In patients with sensitive skins, skin tests should be carried out with the various lotions and adhesives that are commonly used. The stoma therapist should always try to talk to the patient's relatives pre-operatively. They also require a sympathetic listener and careful explanation, as they are often just as anxious as the patient.

Postoperative care

In hospital

The ward staff undertake the early postoperative care, with the stoma therapist playing a supportive role, assisting and advising where necessary. The first appliance should be simple to apply, gentle to the skin, transparent and odour-proof. After this initial period, the patient is shown a few suitable appliances and decides, with the help of the stoma therapist, which appliance to try. The involvement with his own care should be gradual. Initially, the patient just observes while the stoma therapist demonstrates how to change the appliance. Gradually the patient learns how to care for his stoma and change the appliance unaided. If possible, a relative should be familiar with these techniques in case of illness or injury. Details of how to obtain the appliance and, in this country, how to obtain an exemption certificate, are given before the patient is discharged home. He should be sent home with adequate supplies. He should also be told how to contact the stoma therapist in case a problem or emergency arises.

At home

As long as the patient does not live too far away, I feel very strongly that the stoma therapist should make at least one home visit to ensure continuity of care and to ensure that the patient and his relatives are able to cope away from the protective atmosphere of the hospital. When the patient lives too far away, then the district nurse should be asked to visit the patient soon after he returns home and to make further visits as required.

Stoma clinic

On discharge from hospital, every patient should be given an appointment to visit the stoma clinic fairly soon. After this initial visit, he should be seen as often as necessary. Even when everything appears to be going well, stoma patients should be seen at least once a year so that they can be shown any new equipment that has become available. Not only the patients but also their close relatives should always be welcome at the stoma clinic. The clinic should be run on a fairly informal basis so that the patients and their relatives are relaxed and feel able to talk readily about any problems. It is at this stage that particular care should be taken to ensure that the patient has returned to his normal work and social activities. Practical help and encouragement should be given where necessary.

Adolescents have their own problems, as this is a difficult period of adjustment in most people's lives. Add an ileostomy to this situation and it is not surprising that some of them become lonely, depressed and difficult teenagers. It is often helpful to put them in touch with an ileostomist who has already gone through this time. It is also important to keep in close contact with the family to give advice and encouragement.

Other responsibilities of the stoma therapist

Teaching

This is a very important part of the work of a stoma therapist. She has a specialised skill and should teach as many people as possible, both within the hospital and in the community. This aim is best achieved by giving lectures and by giving small groups of people, such as nurses and medical students, practical demonstrations of stoma care on the wards and in the stoma clinic.

Records

Accurate records must be kept for each patient, as this helps to provide good care and produces an efficient filing system to help with research.

Trials

It is important for the stoma therapist to take part in trials to evaluate new products as they become available. This not only keeps the therapist up to date but helps to provide a good service to her patients.

Conclusion

In a world which seems to be obsessed by the body beautiful, the ostomist inevitably feels different. To be effective in minimising this feeling, the stoma therapist must not work alone but must maintain close and effective links with all members of the stoma care team. Our goal must be to help to produce fully integrated and well adjusted ileostomists.

Recommended for further reading

Walker F.C. ed (1976) *Modern Stoma Care.* Churchill-Livingstone, London.
Mahoney J.M. (1976) *Guide to Ostomy Nursing Care.* Little, Brown and Co., Boston.

Chapter 19
The health of ileostomists

H. J. KENNEDY

The first operation to create an ileostomy was performed by J. Y. Brown of St. Louis in the United States of America (Brown, 1913). Several years elapsed before this operation became widely used in the treatment of ulcerative colitis. Strauss was one of the first exponents of this procedure in the United States (Strauss *et al.*, 1924). Some time later, Sir Arthur Hurst, amongst others, described favourable results in patients in England (Hurst, 1940). The next major advance was the development of the first adherent rubber appliance by Koenig, a chemistry student who was a patient of Strauss and Strauss (1944).

In 1951, Gardner and Miller described the operation of ileostomy with simultaneous colectomy or proctocolectomy. Previously, an ileostomy had been formed with later removal of the colon. Gardner and Miller claimed that immediate colectomy or proctocolectomy greatly reduced the mortality and morbidity in their patients. This procedure has since been widely accepted due to the very good results that can be achieved. Another important advance, that helped to improve the health of ileostomists, was the description by Brooke of eversion of the ileostomy stump with primary suture of the mucosa to the skin (Brooke, 1952). This simple technique has considerably reduced the morbidity that previously occurred as a result of scarring and fibrosis of the stoma. Finally, in 1969, Kock described his operation of ileostomy with an intra-abdominal reservoir. This procedure is now performed in some specialist centres and is considered in detail in Chapter 20. Further discussion in the present chapter relates entirely to work undertaken with patients who have a conventional ileostomy. Other advances are taking place in surgery so that, in the future, it may be possible for patients to have the diseased bowel removed without the necessity of an abdominal stoma (Parks and Nicholls, 1978).

Mortality

The mortality related to ileostomy surgery has fallen sharply during the course of the century. The improvement in mortality has occurred for several reasons. First, medical management has improved and the indications for surgery are now well defined. Secondly, surgical techniques have improved, as we have discussed in the introduction. Finally, general advances have taken place in medicine during the past 50 years, such as the development of clinical biochemistry, the introduction of antibiotics and improved anaesthetic techniques.

When considering mortality related to ileostomy surgery, it is best to divide it into immediate mortality, defined as death occurring before the patient leaves hospital, and late mortality, defined as death occurring after the patient returns home.

Immediate mortality

In 1954, Goligher demonstrated that it was possible to reduce the immediate mortality to 2·7% (Table 19.1). The results recorded in this report, when immediate colectomy or proctocolectomy was the operation performed, were in contrast to the results of the previous study of Counsel and Goligher (1952) when the early mortality was 21·6%. In this earlier study, ileostomy alone without immediate colectomy had been the operation performed. Unfortunately, as is shown in Table 19.1, the more recent reports have recorded a higher mortality. Ritchie carried out two studies which showed an early mortality of

Table 19.1. *Mortality related to ileostomy surgery*

	Date	% Mortality	Authors
Immediate mortality	1952	21·6	Counsell & Goligher
	1954	2·7	Goligher
	1966a	11·9	Watts *et al.*
	1968	10·4	Daly
	1972	8·4	Ritchie
	1974	23·7	Ritchie
Late mortality	1968	9	Daly
	1971b	8	Ritchie
	1980	4·6	Goligher

8·1% in St. Mark's hospital and a 23·7% mortality in 34 non-teaching hospitals in the North-East Metropolitan Hospital Region. These figures are particularly disturbing when it is realised that it is possible to have an immediate mortality as low as the 2·7% reported by Goligher and which corresponds to the immediate mortality in Oxford.

Late mortality

The late mortality is also significant, as is shown in Table 19.1. This mortality may be related either to the surgical morbidity (which is discussed later) or to the original disease, especially when a carcinoma is present at the time of operation. As with immediate mortality, it is possible to reduce late mortality to low levels by good medical and surgical management.

General health

The general health of patients surviving ileostomy surgery is very good. This is exemplified by the results of three studies which found that the general health of the patients was good or excellent in 87—96% of cases (Daly, 1968; Watts *et al.*, 1966b; Roy *et al.*, 1970). However there are considerable difficulties encountered by some patients with an ileostomy in relation to surgical morbidity, non-surgical morbidity, and aspects of their psychological, social and sexual life. These factors are discussed in the following sections.

Morbidity related to surgery

Morbidity related to surgery can be considered under several headings: problems with the stoma itself, failure of the perineal wound to heal, and development of intestinal obstruction (Table 19.2). Impairment of sexual function may also be a result of surgery and this is discussed later.

Morbidity related to the stoma

Problems with the stoma have become much less frequent since the introduction of the technique of full-thickness eversion of the ileostomy stump. However, problems still arise and a significant percentage of ileostomy stomas need to be refashioned. There are many reasons why an ileostomy may have to be reconstructed, some of the more common being faulty initial siting of the stoma, ileostomy recession or prolapse, stenosis of the stoma or, occasionally, the development of a parastomal hernia.

Morbidity related to the perineal wound

The figures shown in Table 19.2 are the percentages of patients whose perineal wound has not healed six months after the operation. Even with the more modern technique of primary suture of this wound, one of the most recent reports states that 30% of patients at St. Mark's Hospital have not healed their perineal wound six months after surgery (Marks *et al.*, 1978). The morbidity related to the healing of this wound therefore remains a substantial problem.

Morbidity related to intestinal obstruction

Apart from intestinal obstruction related to the stoma itself, intra-

Table 19.2. *Morbidity related to ileostomy surgery*

	Date	% Morbidity	Authors
Ileostomy requiring refashioning			
	1967	6·0	Daly and Brooke
	1970	8·7	Roy *et al.*
	1971a	10·8	Ritchie
	1980	5·0	Goligher
Perianal wound not healed 6 months after operation			
Open management	1966a	25	Watts *et al.*
	1972	50	Ritchie
Primary suture	1975	30	Irvin and Goligher
	1978	30	Marks *et al.*
Obstruction			
	1966b	8·4	Watts *et al.*
	1967	9·0	Daly and Brooke
	1971a	9·3	Ritchie

abdominal mechanical obstruction not infrequently occurs as a result of ileostomy surgery. The reasons for this include adherence of the small intestine either to the suture line of the pelvic peritoneum or to the laparotomy wound or posterior abdominal wall. Intestinal obstruction may also result from general intra-abdominal adhesions and from strangulation of the small intestine in the para-ileostomy gutter.

General metabolism

General metabolism is thought to be normal in those patients with an ileostomy who have had a minimal resection of small intestine and who do not have Crohn's disease (Table 19.3). Daly found abnormal liver function tests in 4 out of 100 patients, but those patients probably had liver damage associated with ulcerative colitis prior to operation. Other investigators have found normal liver function tests and normal plasma electrolyte levels (Clarke and McKenzie, 1969; Jagenberg *et al.*, 1971; Singer *et al.*, 1973).

Table 19.3. *General metabolism in patients with an ileostomy*

Biochemistry — blood		
urea and electrolytes:	normal	Daly; Clarke and McKenzie; Jagenberg *et al.*; Singer *et al.*
calcium:	normal	Daly; Singer *et al.*
uric acid:	normal	Singer *et al.*
liver function tests:	abnormal in 4	Daly
Haematology		
haemoglobin:	low in 8	Daly
	normal	Clarke and McKenzie; Jagenberg *et al.*
iron and iron-binding capacity:	normal	Jagenberg *et al.*
serum folate:	normal	Jagenberg *et al.*
serum vitamin B_{12}:	normal	Jagenberg *et al.*

Four studies:	Daly (1968)	100 patients
	Clarke and McKenzie (1969)	14 patients
	Jagenberg *et al.* (1971)	10 patients
	Singer *et al.* (1973)	20 patients

Jagenberg and his co-workers found normal haematological values in their patients (Table 19.3). Daly found that 8 out of his 100 patients were anaemic. Four of these patients had menorrhagia, two had cirrhosis of the liver, one had a poor diet and one had unexplained iron-deficiency anaemia.

Absorption and excretion

Apart from salt and water balance, which is discussed in the next section, absorption and excretion of substances in ileostomy patients has not received very much attention. The available data are given in Table 19.4. It is apparent that vitamin B_{12} absorption is normal in the great majority of patients who have not had a terminal ileal resection or suffered from Crohn's disease. Xylose absorption has been found to be marginally low in a few patients, but this finding is unlikely to be of any significance. Protein and fat excretion have both been found to be raised in a number of patients compared to the excretion in normal faeces. This observation is of interest and further work needs to be undertaken in this field.

Water and electrolyte status

For many years salt and water depletion has been a recognised complication of the early postoperative period in patients with an ileostomy.

Table 19.4. *Absorption and excretion in patients with an ileostomy*

| Number of patients | Absorption | | Excretion | | Authors |
	Vit. B_{12}	Xylose	Fat	Protein or faecal nitrogen	
10	1 low	4 low	4 high	–	Jagenberg *et al.* (1971)
15	2 low	2 low	11 high	–	Miettinen and Peltokallio (1971)
10	2 low	–	–	–	Lenz (1976)
5	–	–	–	high	Gibson *et al.* (1976)
16	–	–	normal	high	King *et al.* (1978)

In 1962, Gallagher and his colleagues described episodes of salt and water depletion occurring in patients with well-established ileostomies. Later work suggested that apparently healthy patients with an ileostomy have persistent depletion of sodium and water (Clarke *et al.*, 1967; Hill *et al.*, 1975a). However, in 1978, Turnberg and his co-workers reported that their patients had normal extracellular and total body water volumes, although they did find that total exchangeable sodium and potassium were reduced. As the serum electrolytes were normal in these subjects, they concluded that there must be an intracellular depletion of sodium and potassium.

Another interesting feature of sodium and water balance in patients with an ileostomy is the finding that they probably have an increased potential difference across their ileal mucosa (Isaacs *et al.*, 1976). It is possible that this indicates increased sodium absorption by the mucosa. However, despite evidence for sodium conservation by the kidney and intestine in patients with an ileostomy, plasma aldosterone levels have been found to be normal in almost all cases (Isaacs *et al.*, 1976; Turnberg *et al.*, 1978). As yet, there is no adequate explanation for these interesting observations. Further study is required to try to understand the underlying physiological mechanisms.

Nephrolithiasis

There has been considerable interest in the incidence of nephrolithiasis in patients with an ileostomy. Table 19.5 gives details of the main studies. It should be noted that some of these studies included only those patients whose primary disease had been ulcerative colitis, whereas other studies included patients who had had either ulcerative colitis or Crohn's disease. This may be important when considering the incidence and composition of renal stones in patients with an ileostomy, because Crohn's disease involving the small intestine is known to be associated with an increased incidence of urinary stones (Deren *et al.*, 1962; Gelzayd *et al.*, 1968).

The probable explanation for the increased incidence of urinary stones in Crohn's disease is that malabsorption of fats and the consequent combination of calcium and fatty acids leaves less calcium available for the formation of poorly-soluble calcium oxalate in the intestine (Andersson and Jagenberg, 1974). Therefore the unbound oxalate is absorbed, only to be excreted in high concentrations in the

Table 19.5. *The incidence of nephrolithiasis in patients with an ileostomy*

Number of patients	Disease	% Incidence	Country	Authors
583	UC or Crohn's	7·4	USA	Deren *et al.* (1962)
74	UC	13	Czechoslovakia	Marataka and Nedbal (1964)
79	UC or Crohn's	18	USA	Gelzayd *et al.* (1968)
333	UC	8·4	Australia	Bennett and Hughes (1972)
300	UC	0·7	England (Birmingham)	Alexander (1970)
150	UC	1·3	England (Leeds)	Goligher (1975)
311	UC or Crohn's	4·3	England (London)	Ritchie (1971b)

urine, where it tends to precipitate and form stones. However, more recent work has suggested that patients with steatorrhoea and an ileostomy do not get hyperoxaluria (Dobbins and Binder, 1977; Earnest *et al.*, 1974). The reason for the discrepancy may be that the unbound oxalate is absorbed from the colon in those patients with steatorrhoea and an intact colon (Modigliani *et al.*, 1977).

When patients with ulcerative colitis have been studied, an increased incidence of nephrolithiasis has been found except in England (Alexander, 1970; Goligher, 1980). There is probably about a 1% incidence of urinary stones in the general population in England. In Australia, Bennet and Hughes (1972) found an incidence of 4% in their patients who were being treated medically for ulcerative colitis. After colectomy and the formation of an ileostomy, this incidence increased to 8·4%. A high incidence of nephrolithiasis has also been reported from the United States of America and from Czechoslovakia.

The composition of the stones found in patients with an ileostomy is unknown in most cases. However, there appears to be a higher than normal incidence of uric acid calculi (Deren *et al.*, 1962; Maratka and Nedbal, 1964; Bennett and Hughes, 1972). The factors favouring the formation of uric acid stones in patients with an ileostomy are reduced urine output and increased urinary acidity. Probably, there is also an increased incidence of calcium-containing stones (Grossman and Nugent, 1967). This is an interesting field of study and we have much more to learn.

Cholelithiasis

An increased incidence of cholelithiasis in patients with ileal disfunction has been well documented (Heaton and Read, 1969; Cohen *et al.*, 1971; Dowling *et al.*, 1972). The situation with regard to patients with an ileostomy is less certain. Hill and his colleagues found a 24·5% incidence of gall-stones in a study of 108 patients with an ileostomy (Hill *et al.*, 1975b). They estimated that this incidence was about three times that expected in a sample of the general population of similar age and sex. On analysis of their data, they found that the incidence of gall-stones was high in those patients whose primary disease was Crohn's disease or who had had more than 10 cm of the terminal ileum removed. They found no increased incidence in those patients who had had less than 10 cm of terminal ileum removed and whose primary disease was ulcerative colitis. However, a study from Cardiff reports a 20% incidence in a group of 55 patients, all of whom had had ulcerative colitis and in whom less than 10 cm of terminal ileum had been removed (Jones *et al.*, 1976).

Loss of functioning terminal ileum due to either resection or disease is known to impair the enterohepatic circulation (Heaton and Read, 1969; Cohen *et al.*, 1971; Dowling *et al.*, 1972). This results in loss of bile salts and consequently in an increased incidence of cholelithiasis. Normal absorption of bile salts and a normal bile-salt pool have been found in patients with an ileostomy (Percy-Robb *et al.*, 1969; Morris *et al.*, 1973). Therefore, it would be surprising to find an increased incidence of gall-stones in all types of patients with an ileostomy. If the high incidence found by Jones and his co-workers is confirmed, then it must be presumed that the colon does, in fact, play a significant role in bile salt metabolism.

Social and psychological aspects

There have been three major surveys of the social and psychological effects of an ileostomy (Daly, 1968; Watts *et al.*, 1966b; Roy *et al.*, 1970). The main findings are shown in Table 19.6.

Work

The great majority of patients return to their normal full-time occupation. In the very few patients in whom a change in occupation may be advisable, such as those engaged in very heavy manual labour, some help and advice may be required. This subject is discussed in more detail in Chapter 18.

Diet

As can be seen from Table 19.6, most patients eat a normal diet. The usual recommendation is to take care initially when eating poorly-

Table 19.6. *Social and psychological aspects of life with an ileostomy*

1 Work	95%	full-time work	Daly
	96%	full-time work	Watts *et al.*
	95·6%	full-time work	Roy *et al.*
2 Diet	83%	entirely normal	Daly
	17%	avoided nuts, fruits, skins etc.	
	65·7%	normal	Roy *et al.*
	34·3%	minor restrictions, often to control weight	
3 Social activities	no limitation except golf		Daly
	93·5%	normal	Watts *et al.*
	82%	normal	Roy *et al.*
	18%	limited by bathroom facilities and noise from ileostomy	
	17%	discontinued sports, mainly contact sports	

Three studies:	Daly	(1968)	—	100 patients interviewed
	Watts *et al.*	(1966b)	—	119 patients interviewed
	Roy *et al.*	(1970)	—	344 patients given questionnaire

digested foods, such as nuts, fruits, skins and sweetcorn. Patients are advised to try these foods in small quantities at first and always to chew them thoroughly before swallowing. There are few problems when this advice is followed. Some other foods, such as onions and mushrooms, can cause diarrhoea and the passage of more flatus than usual. As found by Roy and his colleagues, many patients with an ileostomy find that they tend to put on too much weight and they may have to restrict their calorie intake.

Social activities

The large majority of patients return to their normal social activities. Daly found that some of his patients had difficulty in playing golf, as the twisting of the body tended to loosen the appliance. With more recent equipment, such as stomahesive and light-weight bags, this is seldom a problem. Patients are generally advised to avoid violent contact sports, such as rugby football, but otherwise they are encouraged to be as active as possible. Daly found that the activities of his patients included under-water swimming, gliding, camping and dancing.

Sexual aspects

The results of four studies of the sexual function of patients with an ileostomy is summarised in Table 19.7. The way in which the questions are asked is an important factor in any research involving sexual function. It can be seen in the table that, in three out of the four studies, each patient was personally interviewed, whereas, in the remaining study, the patients were sent a questionnaire. The mode of questioning may be very important in determining the results of the research. For instance, in the study in which patients were sent a questionnaire it can be seen in the table that a high incidence of sexual difficulties was found, particularly in female patients. It is difficult to be certain which form of questioning gives the more accurate information in this sensitive field. Nevertheless, there are some important points which emerge from these studies.

Male sexual function

Table 19.7 shows the proportion of patients who have either total or

H. J. Kennedy

Table 19.7. *Sexual aspects of life with an ileostomy*

Number of patients	Form of questions	Male % impaired	Female		Authors
			Intercourse	% Impaired fertility	
100 m 62 f	interview	11·0	–	reduced	Daly (1968)
41 m 67 f	interview	27	7·5	–	Watts *et al.* (1966b)
118 m 165 f	questionnaire	29	33	–	Burnham *et al.* (1977)
67 m 40 f	interview	22	1·75	reduced	Grüner *et al.* (1977)

m = male   f = female

partial loss of sexual function. This very high rate of sexual impairment is of great concern, particularly as many of the patients are young. In two of the studies, sexual potency in male patients with an ileostomy and panproctocolectomy is compared with the potency in patients who either have an ileostomy with the rectum remaining or have had an ileo-rectal anastomosis (Burnham *et al.*, 1977; Grüner *et al.*, 1977). In both of these studies it was found that the sexual function of male patients was normal when the rectum was left in place. Therefore, the high rate of sexual impairment in males appears to be directly related to the removal of the rectum. There is a very low rate of impotence in men who have a panproctocolectomy in Oxford. We believe that this is because of the technique of perimuscular excision of the rectum which is described in Chapter 16.

Female sexual function

The information concerning female sexual function is less precise. Table 19.7 shows the markedly different results in relation to female dysfunction found in the various studies. Some of these patients complain of loss of libido because they have lost normal sensation in the perineum. However, the common cause of sexual dysfunction in these women is dyspareunia.

Fertility is probably reduced in female ileostomists (Daly, 1968;

Grüner *et al.*, 1977). This may result either from inflammation in the pelvis due to the diseased colon and rectum or from adhesions and scarring following surgery. Daly suggested that primarily closure of the pelvic peritoneum might reduce the incidence of female infertility following surgery.

There seems to be a very low incidence of physical difficulties due to the stoma during sexual intercourse (Burnham *et al.*, 1977). Some ileostomists find that it is helpful to fix the appliance by wearing a girdle or other suitable garment. With regard to emotional reactions to the stoma, Burnham and his colleagues found that half of their patients felt less attractive sexually, although only 9% of wives and 6% of husbands shared this view. Grüner and his co-workers found that extra-marital activity was low in both their female and male patients with an ileostomy. However, they found that coital frequency was normal in their married patients.

There is no doubt that some patients with an ileostomy experience significant sexual problems. These difficulties may be minimised by good surgical technique and by good counselling from the medical staff treating each patient.

Conclusions

The aim of this chapter has been to summarise the current state of knowledge concerning the health of patients with an ileostomy. It is apparent that good results can be obtained if skilled teams of doctors and nurses care for these patients. Unfortunately the results that are being achieved at the moment are by no means optimal. It is also apparent that we have much to learn concerning both the metabolic consequences and the social, psychological and sexual aspects of life with an ileostomy.

References

Alexander F.G. (1970) Quoted by Ritchie (1971b).
Andersson H. and Jagenberg R. (1974) *Gut,* **15**, 360.
Bennett R.C. and Hughes E.S.R. (1972) *Brit. med. J.* **ii**, 494.
Brooke B.N. (1952) *Lancet,* **ii**, 102.
Brown J.Y. (1913) *Surg. Gynec. Obstet.* **16**, 610.
Burnham W.R., Lennard-Jones J.E. and Brooke B.N. (1977) *Gut,* **18**, 673.
Clarke A.M. and McKenzie R.G. (1969) *Lancet,* **ii**, 395.

Clarke A.M., Chirnside A., Hill G.L. and Pope G. (1967) *Lancet,* **ii**, 740.

Cohen S., Kaplan M., Gottlieb C. and Patterson J. (1971) *Gastroenterology,* **60**, 237.

Counsell P.B. and Goligher J.C. (1952) *Lancet,* **2**, 1045.

Daly D.W. (1968) *Ann. Roy. Coll. Surg.* **42**, 38.

Daly D.W. and Brooke B.N. (1967) *Lancet,* **2**, 62.

Deren J.J., Porush J.G., Levitt M.F. and Khilnani M.T. (1962) *Ann. Intern. Med.* **56**, 843.

Dobbins J.W. and Binder H.J. (1977) *New Engl. J. Med.* **296**, 298.

Dowling R.H., Bell G.D. and White J. (1972) *Gut,* **13**, 415.

Earnest D.L., Johnson G., Williams D.E. and Admirand W. (1974) *Gastroenterology,* **66**, 1114.

Gallagher N.D., Harrison D.D. and Skyring A.P. (1962) *Gut,* **3**, 219.

Gardner C. and Miller G.G. (1951) *Arch. Surg.* **63**, 370.

Gelzayd E.A., Breuer R.I. and Kirsner J.B. (1968) *Amer. J. dig. Dis.* **13**, 1027.

Gibson J.A., Sladen G.E. and Dawson A.M. (1976) *Brit. J. Nutr.* **35**, 61.

Goligher J.C. (1954) *Ann. Roy. Coll. Surg.* **8**, 421.

Goligher J.C. (1980) *Surgery of the anus, rectum and colon* 4 e. Bailliere Trindall. London.

Grossman M.S. and Nugent F.W. (1967) *Amer. J. dig. Dis.* **12**, 491.

Grüner O.P.N., Naas R., Fretheim B. and Gjone E. (1977) *Scand. J. Gastroenterol.* **12**, 193.

Heaton K.W. and Read A.E. (1969) *Brit. med. J.* **iii**, 494.

Hill G.L., Goligher J.C., Smith A.H. and Mair W.S.J. (1975a). *Brit. J. Surg.* **62**, 524.

Hill G.L., Mair W.S.J. and Goligher J.C. (1975b) *Gut,* **16**, 932.

Hurst A.F. (1940) *Proc. roy. Soc. Med.* **33**, 645.

Irvin T.T. and Goligher J.C. (1975) *Brit. J. Surg.* **62**, 749.

Isaacs P.E.T., Horth C.E. and Turnberg L.A. (1976) *Gastroenterology,* **70**, 52.

Jagenberg R., Dotevall G., Kewenter J., Kock N.G. and Philipson B. (1971) *Gut,* **12**, 437.

Jones M.R., Gregory D., Evans K.T. and Rhodes J. (1976) *Clin. Radiol.* **27**, 561.

King R.F.G.J., Millward S. and Hill G.L. (1978) *Gut,* **19**, A456.

Kock N.G. (1969) *Arch. Surg.* **99**, 223.

Lenz K. (1976) *Scand. J. Gastroenterol.* **11**, 769.

Maratka Z. and Nedbal J. (1964) *Gut,* **5**, 3.

Marks C.G., Ritchie J.K. Todd I.P. and Wadsworth J. (1978) *Brit. J. Surg.* **65**, 560.

Miettinen T.A. and Peltokallio P. (1971) *Scand. J. Gastroenterol.* **6**, 543.

Modigliani R., Labayle D., Aymes C. and Denvil R. (1978) *Scand. J. Gastroenterol.* **113**, 187.

Morris J.S., Low-Beer T.S. and Heaton K.W. (1973) *Scand. J. Gastroenterol.* **8**, 424.

Parks A.G. and Nicholls R.J. (1978) *Brit. med. J.* **2**, 85.

Percy-Robb I.W., Jalan K.N., McManus J.P.A. and Sircus W. (1969) *Brit. J. Surg.* **56**, Abs. 96, 694.

Ritchie J.K. (1971a) *Gut,* **12**, 528.

Ritchie J.K. (1971b) *Gut,* **12**, 536.

Ritchie J.K. (1972) *Brit. J. Surg.* **59**, 345.

Ritchie J.K. (1974) *Brit. med. J.* **i**, 264.

Roy P.H., Saver W.G., Beahrs O.H. and Farrow G.M. (1970) *Amer. J. Surg.* **119**, 77.

Singer A.M., Bennett R.C., Carter N.G. and Hughes E.S.R. (1973) *Brit. med. J.* **iii**, 141.

Strauss A.A., Friedman J. and Block L. (1924) *Surg. Clin. N. Amer.* **4**, 667.

Strauss A.A. and Strauss S.F. (1944) *Surg. Clin. N. Amer.* **24**, 211.

Turnberg L.A., Morris A.I., Hawker P.C., Herman K.J., Shields R.A. and Horth C.E. (1978) *Gut,* **19**, 563.

Watts J. McK., De Dombal F.T. and Goligher J.C. (1966a) *Brit. J. Surg.* **53**, 1005.

Watts J. McK., De Dombal F.T. and Goligher J.C. (1966b) *Brit. J. Surg.* **53**, 1014.

Chapter 20
Continent ileostomy

NILS G. KOCK

To eliminate the problems associated with a conventional ileostomy, the so called 'continent ileostomy' was elaborated and devised for clinical use in 1967 in Göteborg, Sweden. In this type of ileostomy, a low-pressure ileal pouch is constructed from the terminal ileum for collection and storage of the intestinal discharge. The outlet of the pouch is provided with an intussusception valve which prevents involuntary leakage through the ileostomy (Fig. 20.1). The patients empty the pouch when convenient 3–4 times a day by intubation and in the meantime the ileostomy is covered only by a small compress.

An account of the evolution of this type of ileostomy, including operative details, has been given by Kock *et al.* (1977).

Patients and results

In January 1980 the total group comprised 314 patients. The great majority of the patients had been operated upon because of ulcerative colitis but 50 patients with Crohn's disease are also included (Table 20.1). Roughly 50% of the patients were provided with the continent ileostomy at the time of performing proctocolectomy whereas, in the other patients, a conventional ileostomy was converted to a continent ileostomy at a second operation.

Seven patients have died from complications connected to the operation, which means a 2·2% operative mortality rate. Non-fatal major complications necessitating surgical intervention have occurred in 48 patients (16%) and include peritonitis or abscesses due to anastomotic leak in 13 cases, intestinal obstruction or suspicion of obstruction in 17 cases, and wound dehiscence in six patients.

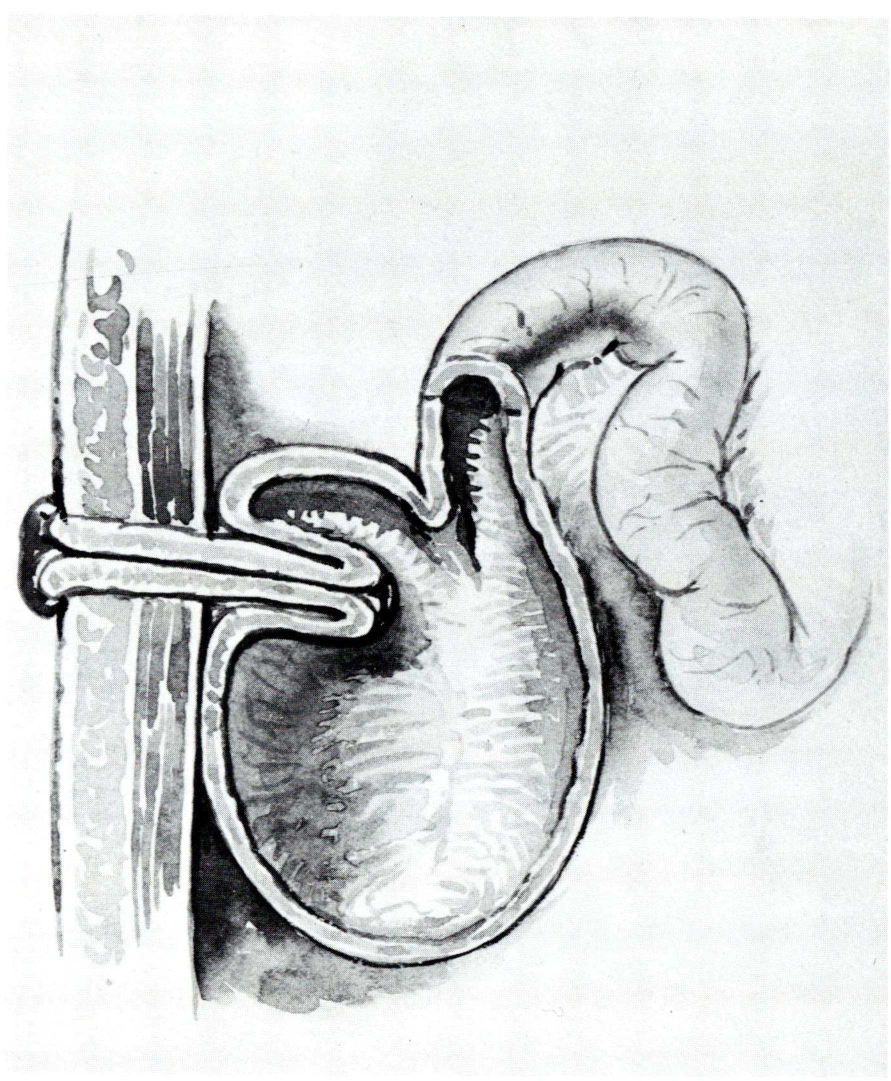

Fig. 20.1. *Schematic drawing of the ileostomy reservoir in situ.*

Table 20.1. *Diagnoses in 314 patients provided with a continent ileostomy*

Type of disease	Number of patients
Ulcerative colitis	242
Crohn's disease	50
Polyposis	17
Miscellaneous	5
Total	314

When the material was analyzed at follow-up, it was found that six patients had died of causes not related to the operation and that 14 reservoirs had been removed for various reasons. There were, thus, 287 patients available for evaluation of the functional results. The functional results were evaluated in terms of the need for the patient to wear an ileostomy appliance. Out of the 287 patients, 276 never used an appliance (96%). Of the patients with a nipple valve, 97% had excellent functional results (Table 20.2).

Late complications

The present results have not been achieved without difficulty. In order to achieve permanent continence, surgical correction of the nipple valve has been necessary in a great number of patients. Construction of the intussusception valve creates a weak point on the mesenteric side by

Table 20.2. *Functional results in 287 patients with a continent ileostomy*

	Number of patients	Always	Ileostomy appliance Occasionally	Never
Without nipple valve	29	1	3	25 (85%)
With nipple valve	258	3	4	251 (97%)
Total	287	4	7	276 (96%)

wedging fat and peritoneal blood vessels between the intestinal walls forming the nipple. When the reservoir starts to dilate, the mesentery is stretched and starts to pull on the nipple valve, and it tries to reduce the nipple valve on the mesenteric side. Simultaneously, the nipple valve is dislocated to the mesenteric side, making insertion of the catheter difficult.

In order to prevent sliding of the nipple valve, the operative technique for construction of the nipple valve has been modified several times. At present, a simplified method is under evaluation. By use of the GIA instrument, 4 rows of staples are applied longitudinally on the intussusception valve and the base of the nipple valve is secured by a sling of fascia or Marlex mesh threaded through an opening in the mesentery and encircling the base of the nipple. So far, no sliding has occurred in 32 patients operated upon with this technique and these results should be compared to the sliding incidence of 46 and 22% with previous methods. The observation time for the patients operated upon with the latest modification is still relatively short but we feel that this technique is very promising.

It is true that construction of a continent ileostomy has been afflicted with a relatively high incidence of complications. However, growing experience and modification of the technique have markedly diminished the complication rate (Table 20.3).

Patients with Crohn's disease

In our group, 50 patients with Crohn's disease are included. In some of these patients, the preoperative diagnosis was ulcerative colitis, but later turned out to be Crohn's disease. Some further patients with Crohn's

Table 20.3. *Operative mortality and complication rate during two consecutive time periods*

Time period	Operative mortality	Major complications
1967–1974	7/162 (4%)	37/155 (24%)
1975–1979	0/152 (0%)	11/152 (7%)
Total	7/314 (2%)	48/307 (16%)

disease strictly limited to the colon were also selected for the procedure. When the results were analyzed, we found that the incidence of major operative complications for patients with Crohn's disease was twice as high as for the other group of patients. Furthermore, eight reservoirs had been removed from a total of 49 patients with Crohn's disease whereas only six reservoirs had been removed from a total of 236 patients with ulcerative colitis. The reasons for removal of the reservoirs in patients with Crohn's disease were operative complications in two patients, recurrence of the disease in the pouch in four patients, and late complications, such as fistulae, in two patients.

Recurrence has been recorded in 17 of the 49 patients with Crohn's disease. In five patients, the recurrence was located in the reservoir, in six it was proximal to the reservoir and in six patients the recurrence involved the reservoir as well as the bowel proximal to the reservoir. In four of the patients the reservoir was removed, in ten patients a small bowel resection was performed and in three patients no surgical removal of the diseased intestine has so far been performed. At follow up, 11 patients had been lost from the series, three had died and in eight patients the reservoir had been removed. Thirty nine patients were left for evaluation of the functional results and 34 (87%) of these never used ileostomy appliances.

Despite the good functional results obtained in a proportion of the patients with Crohn's disease, we feel that our figures suggest that patients with this disease should only exceptionally be provided with a continent ileostomy.

Bacteriology, morphology and absorption

The reservoir procedure makes use of a considerable length of the terminal ileum and creates a blind loop. Invasion of bacteria into this type of intestinal pouch in unavoidable and the resulting change in the micro-flora could theoretically affect the mucous membrane of the reservoir as well as impairing absorption. In order to investigate the possible biological consequences of the ileostomy reservoir, a number of studies have been performed in patients with this type of ileostomy. With regard to the number of microorganisms, the reservoir contents occupy an intermediate position between the conventional ileostomy discharge and normal faeces. Also, with regard to the ratio of anaerobes and aerobes, the reservoir contents are intermediate. There is thus an increased number of microorganisms and anaerobic dominance in the reservoir (Brandberg *et al.*, 1972).

In order to study the morphology of the mucous membrane, biopsies were obtained from the reservoirs in six patients at monthly intervals over a period of one year and then in the same patients after two and eight years. One month after operation, the villous height was significantly decreased in the reservoir mucous·membrane. After this initial decrease, the villous height slowly increased throughout the study period of six to ten years but still differed significantly from the control material at the end of the study period. Under the electron microscope, no signs of intracellular changes in the epithelial cells were found and the brush border layer remained intact (Philipson *et al.*, 1975). The enzymatic activity of the epithelial cells did not differ from control material.

These studies have therefore demonstrated that the ileal mucosa of the intestinal segment used for construction of the reservoir undergoes a transformation characterized by increased cell turnover and decreased villous height. However, this process is not progressive and the epithelial covering remains intact and maintains its enzymatic activity.

The absorption of fat, bile salts and vitamin B_{12} was studied in 14 proctocolectomized patients 6–10 years after construction of a continent ileostomy (Nilsson *et al.*, 1979). All patients were in excellent health and displayed no signs of malnutrition. Schilling test disclosed subnormal absorption of vitamin B_{12} in one patient and borderline values in five. However, none of these patients showed subnormal plasma levels of vitamin B_{12}.

Faecal fat excretion was increased in two patients but without any clinical signs of fat malabsorption. The mean weight of the intestinal discharge during a high-fat diet period was 830 g per 24 hours. The mean faecal excretion of ^{14}C-cholic acid was 46% in the reservoir group, compared with 18% in the group with conventional ileostomies during a 24-hour period. There was no correlation between the cholic acid excretion and the faecal fat excretion.

Although borderline values for the Schilling tests were found in some patients and faecal loss of bile acids was increased in most of the patients, the metabolic consequences of the ileal pouch do not seem to differ significantly from those of a conventional ileostomy. The excellent health of patients 6–10 years after construction of the ileal pouch indicates that the ileal pouch as such does not cause serious metabolic disturbances or malabsorption.

Quality of life

In order to elucidate the influence of the continent ileostomy on the quality of life, studies were performed on two groups of patients. Ten patients who had had a well-functioning conventional ileostomy were questioned after conversion to a continent ileostomy. After conversion, they all discovered that, with the conventional ileostomy, they had lacked confidence and that the conventional ileostomy had restricted their working capacity as well as their leisure activity and sexual life. Most of these problems were eliminated after conversion (Table 20.4). In another study, 40 patients with ulcerative colitis who had undergone conversion from a conventional ileostomy to a continent ileostomy were questioned about the influence of the different types of ileostomy on sexual function. With the conventional ileostomy, four out of 13 men (31%) and 14 out of 26 women (50%) considered their sexual activity to have been reduced. After conversion all but one woman regarded their sexual activity as normal. There have been ten pregnancies among our patients and in every case delivery has occurred without complication.

It is thus evident that the continent ileostomy offers the patients a quality of life superior to that with a conventional ileostomy. The excellent health of the majority of patients with this type of ileostomy, some of them now having been observed for up to 12 years, and the results of studies of the biological consequences of the ileostomy reservoir indicate that favourable effects can be expected in patients

Table 20.4. *The influence of the type of ileostomy on some aspects of life in 10 patients who were converted from a conventional to a continent ileostomy*

	Conventional ileostomy	Continent ileostomy
Restricted working capacity	7	0
Restricted leisure activity	10	2
Problems in sex life	5	1
Lack of confidence	10	0

correctly selected for this procedure. We believe that the continent ileostomy procedure now has a definite place in ileostomy surgery.

ACKNOWLEDGEMENT

I am grateful to my colleagues, Dr Helge E. Myrvold and Dr Lars O. Nilsson, for permission to include some unpublished data in this chapter.

References

Brandberg Å., Kock N.G. and Philipson B. (1972) *Gastroenterology,* **63**, 413.
Kock N.G., Darle N., Hultén L., Kewenter J., Myrvold H. and Philipson B. (1977) Current Problems in Surgery, Vol. XIV, No. 8.
Nilsson L.O., Andersson J., Hultén L., Jagenberg R., Kock N.G., Myrvold H.E. and Philipson B. (1979) *Gut,* **20**, 499.
Philipson B., Brandberg Å., Jagenberg R., Kock N.G., Lager I. and Åhrén C. (1975) *Scand. J. Gastroenterol.* **10**, 145.

Chapter 21
Ileo-rectal anastomosis

PETER F. JONES

Many thousands of patients have now had their lives saved, or made worthwhile, by proctocolectomy with spout ileostomy. The outstanding merit of this operation (especially in ulcerative colitis) is that it is reliable and effective, allowing the patient to regain health and strength quickly, to set about living a full life, and to return to regular work. After the first few months there is usually little need for regular hospital supervision. This is the yardstick by which other surgical methods of treating inflammatory bowel disease must be judged, and it is quite an exacting one.

However, colitis often occurs in young people, and to them an ileostomy is a very unwelcome part of their treatment. It is therefore hardly surprising that surgeons have tried to avoid a continuously active stoma on the abdominal wall and there are now a number of operations which aim to circumvent this problem in one way or another (Table 21.1). Ileo-rectal anastomosis, following removal of the whole colon, was the first of these operations to be tried, nearly 80 years ago, and the purpose of this paper is to make a detailed review of personal and collective experience of this operation.

Personal series

Between 1958 and 1979 a total of 112 patients underwent total colectomy for ulcerative colitis or Crohn's colitis (Table 21.2). Throughout this period, it was the consistent policy of the author to preserve the rectum and perform ileo-rectal anastomosis whenever this appeared to be feasible. In the event, 58 patients (51%) had a proctocolectomy with spout ileostomy (9 having the rectal excision performed at a second

Table 21.1. *Operations for proctocolitis which avoid spout ileostomy*

Total colectomy with ileo-rectal anastomosis (Lilienthal, 1901)

Total colectomy, excision of rectal mucosa and anal ileostomy (Ravitch and Handelsman, 1951)

Proctocolectomy and continent ileostomy (Kock, 1969)

Subtotal excision of colon and rectum with caecal pull-through (Hughes and Bennett, 1972)

Subtotal colectomy and caecoproctostomy (Webster and Howard, 1973)

Proctocolectomy, ileal pouch and ileoanal anastomosis (Parks and Nicholls, 1978)

---

stage). The 10 patients who had a total colectomy only were all deemed unfit for rectal excision and the 5 who died were all emergency colectomies for perforations with peritonitis or for megacolon.

Forty-five patients (40%) were selected pre-operatively as being suitable for ileo-rectal anastomosis, 43 having this operation at the same time as total colectomy; the other two had an emergency total colectomy and ileostomy, and the ileo-rectal anastomosis was performed later. The criteria which were used to choose candidates for ileo-rectal anastomosis were:

(a) the anal canal looked and felt normal.

(b) the rectum was not more than mildly inflamed and appeared to have supple, distensible walls.

(c) in a borderline case, anastomosis was chosen when the patient was below 25 years of age or if the patient strongly preferred this operation.

In three patients we were influenced towards anastomosis by the personality or social circumstances of the patient. One patient whose severe proctitis would normally have justified rectal excision had a religious objection to blood transfusion and it was therefore thought wise not to attempt to remove the rectum. The need for continued annual follow-up with sigmoidoscopy was explained to the patients.

These criteria were not consciously varied over the twenty years, and

Table 21.2. *Total colectomy for colitis. (Personal series 1958–79)*

	Total	Emergency	Deaths
Proctocolectomy			
One-stage	48	12	1
Two-stage	9	8	0
Total colectomy			
Rectum not removed	6	6	5
Hartmann's procedure	4	2	0
Total colectomy and			
Ileo-rectal anastomosis	45	1	2
Total	112	29	8*

*(7 emergency)

pre-operative knowledge, by rectal or colonic biopsy, of Crohn s colitis did not affect the decision, which was always made on the general features of the rectum and anal canal. Details of the 45 patients are summarised in Table 21.3.

Surgical technique

Total colectomy was carried out by standard methods. Whenever possible, only 1–2 cm of ileum adjacent to the ileo-caecal valve were excised; 8 patients had between 10 and 30 cm of diseased ileum removed, 3 of these having Crohn's disease. In each patient, after mobilising the whole colon, the rectum was divided opposite the sacral promontory and the rectal mucosa inspected. If severe granularity or ulceration were seen, a further length of rectum was resected until normal or near-normal rectum was reached, and in 4 patients this led to the rectum being divided at 9, 11, 12 and 12 cm from the anus. The inferior mesenteric and superior rectal arteries were not ligated. An end-to-end anastomosis was made in every case (using continuous chromic catgut during the first 12 years, and thereafter interrupted all-coats mattress sutures of silk or nurolon). The mesenteric gap was closed. In no case was a protective ileostomy formed above the anastomosis.

Table 21.3. *Details of 45 patients having ileo-rectal anastomosis*

	Total	UC	Crohn's
		Histology	
Sex			
Male	20	17	3
Female	25	20	5
Ages			
At school (8–17 years)	12	10	2
Young adult (18–30 years)	19	15	4
Over 30 years	14	12	2
	45	37	8

Results

Forty three patients made a good initial recovery and the anastomosis healed uneventfully. Two patients died, one being the only patient to have an ileo-rectal anastomosis made in conjunction with an emergency total colectomy; the anastomosis leaked on the seventh day, a loop ileostomy was made on the following day but the patient died from progressive sepsis on the fourteenth day. The other patient had to be re-opened for adhesive obstruction on the eighth day and died two weeks later from uncontrolled sepsis. (Both these deaths occurred over 15 years ago and we have never again considered doing an ileo-rectal anastomosis at the time of emergency colectomy).

Among the 43 survivors of operation, three required a laparotomy for adhesive small bowel obstruction within three weeks of colectomy, and in one the bowel was so stuck to the anastomosis that this had to be taken down and a terminal ileostomy formed; because of progressive sclerosing cholangitis this patient has never been fit for re-anastomosis. One patient developed a lung abscess, one a peri-anal abscess, one a subphrenic abscess and one a residual abdominal abscess, all save the lung abscess needing drainage. There were no other major problems during convalescence. It usually took 4–5 days for the small bowel to become active after operation and then many patients passed fairly loose frequent stools but this usually settled quickly. It is most unusual for anyone to be incontinent and this has not occurred after discharge from hospital.

Progress after discharge

This section must be divided into three sections — those who have required late excision of the rectum, those who have subsequently died, and those who have survived with the ileo-rectal anastomosis intact.

(a) Six of the 45 patients have required subsequent ileostomy (Table 21.4) and in 5 the rectum had to be excised for progressive proctitis. In two patients this had to be done quickly when an ileo-rectal anastomosis which had given a good result for two years was suddenly complicated by an episode of acute proctitis; one patient presented with severe rectal haemorrhage and the other with a rapidly progressive relapse with bacteraemia. Both these patients required very vigorous resuscitation with urgent rectal excision, and have since been very well. The other three patients went more slowly downhill, suffering increasing disability from very active proctitis with deep ulceration, and all were greatly improved by rectal excision.

(b) Late deaths are detailed in Table 21.5. The three patients who

Table **21.4**. *Outcome: total colectomy + ileo-rectal anastomosis*

45 patients

Conversion to ileostomy

Sex	Age at operation	Interval	Reason for conversion
F	30	12 days	Laparotomy for intestinal obstruction. Sclerosing cholangitis
F	22	2 years	Severe rectal haemorrhage
M	20	2 years	Recurrent disease (Died 11 years — renal failure)
F	19	2 years	Proctitis — Bacteraemia
M	16	3 years	Crohn's disease. Anal fistulae (Died 7 years — Crohn's disease)
M	23	7 years	Progressive proctitis

Ileo-rectal anastomosis intact at present in 32 patients

Table 21.5. *Outcome: total colectomy + ileo-rectal anastomosis*

45 patients

Operative deaths   2 — Emergency operation. Leak at 7 days. Death sepsis 23 days.

— Intestinal obstruction 6 days. Death sepsis 19 days

Late deaths

Sex	Age at operation	Survival	Cause of death
F	40	5 months	Anorexia nervosa
M	17	6 months	Hepatic metastases, Ca coli
M	17	8 years	Chronic active hepatitis
M	54	10 years	'Natural causes'
M	65	14 years	Carcinoma oesophagus

lived for 8–14 years all had good results from their ileo-rectal anastomoses. The youth who already had hepatic metastases at the time of anastomosis had very useful palliation during the short period that he survived. The fifth patient developed chronic active hepatitis 6 years after his ileo-rectal anastomosis, having been very well and asymptomatic throughout that time, with only very mild inflammation in the rectum. He died in liver failure 2 years after the onset of hepatitis.

(c) The 32 survivors have been carefully reviewed at an annual follow-up examination, although one has been lost to follow-up after 14 years of supervision and one patient has consistently refused to have a sigmoidoscopy since operation. Adhesive intestinal obstruction arose after several years in 4 patients and one required three operations for this reason (on the last occasion, 3 years ago, intestinal intubation (Munro and Jones, 1978) was performed and she has been very well since). One patient with ankylosing spondylitis before operation has had very little trouble since, one patient suffered with joint effusions for 2 years after operation but has had no trouble for the past 8 years, and one patient had erythema nodosum for 2 years after operation but has had no trouble in the past 6 years.

Bowel frequency and the appearance of the rectal mucosa on sigmoidoscopy are recorded in Tables 21.6 and 21.7. All 31 patients recently

Table 21.6. *Ileo-rectal anastomosis*

Stool Frequency/ 24 hours	
1—3	14
4—5	15
6—7	3
	32

reviewed are in good general health and are able to lead normal lives, doing their usual work, and running their homes. Three of the women have married and have borne children since operation and a fourth has had further children since the operation. There has been no disturbance of sexual function among the males.

Generally speaking, bowel frequency has tended to improve with the passage of time. A few have had problems with proctitis in the first year or two after operation but these have been controlled with standard treatment and only two use sulphasalazine tablets regularly.

Care is taken to obtain biopsy specimens of the rectal mucosa at each follow-up visit and these have been examined by an experienced histologist for evidence of dysplasia, so far with no evidence of such change. The great majority of patients show inflammatory changes in the mucosa but these bear little relation to the functional result. It is quite common for some stenosis of the ano-rectal ring to occur and often the interphalangeal joint of the index finger is gripped on digital examination.

Table 21.7. *Ileo-rectal anastomosis*

Degree of inflammation in rectum at sigmoidoscopy		
Grade 1	(Normal)	9
Grade 2	(Mild)	18
Grade 3	(Moderate)	3
Grade 4	(Severe)	0

No biopsy evidence of dysplasia

This does not make it difficult to pass the 1·5 cm sigmoidoscope and there have been no symptoms from this narrowing. The consistency of the stool in the rectum varies to a remarkable degree, some patients having a thick porridgy stool while in others there is a green watery fluid: this difference is not related to the state of the rectal mucosa.

No distinction has been drawn in this review of late results between patients who had ulcerative colitis and the eight who had Crohn's colitis. Among these eight, one had to have a rectal excision and ileostomy for progressive rectal disease 3 years after anastomosis and this patient died after a further 4 years from the spread of Crohn's disease into the whole length of the small intestine. Of the other 7 patients, 5 have 1–3 stools per day, 2 have 4–5 stools per day. They are all leading normal lives and, so far, show no evidence of recurrent disease.

Discussion

Before summarising the results obtained by surgeons who use ileo-rectal anastomosis, there are three special aspects which require discussion.

Carcinoma of the rectal stump

This is, and must remain, the major deterrent to the use of ileo-rectal anastomosis in ulcerative colitis and requires the most careful analysis. The development of a carcinoma in the rectum differs from recurrent proctitis in two major ways:

(a) The patient is quickly aware of progressive or recurrent inflammation in the rectal stump but there are no characteristic symptoms of carcinomatous change. Considerable care is needed to detect an early curable carcinoma even at sigmoidoscopy.

(b) If late proctitis gives enough trouble, the rectum can be excised, with minimal mortality, and the patient can thereafter lead a healthy life. When a carcinoma develops in the rectal stump it is characteristically of high malignancy and the majority of patients have not so far survived this complication, even with radical rectal excision.

On the other hand, it is important to place neoplastic change in its correct place and, serious though it is to the individual, it is a rare complication. Until recently there were only scattered reported cases but the analysis by Baker *et al.* (1978) of Mr. Stanley Aylett's unique series of ileo-rectal anastomoses, from the Gordon Hospital, has allowed much the most extensive examination of the problem to be published (Table 21.8). There were 374 survivors of total colectomy for ulcerative colitis available for examination, of whom 22 developed a carcinoma in the rectal stump. Of these, 18 were poorly differentiated neoplasms and only 6 of them survive, 3 being still within a year of operation. Nothing could more clearly underline the gravity of this complication. The following facts emerge from this survey.

(1) Aylett (1976) himself suggests that some of these tumours arose in strictured rectums, which he preserved during the earlier part of his

Table 21.8. *Ileo-rectal anastomosis*

		Carcinoma in the Rectal Stump			
Authors	Patients with IRA	Patients with carcinoma rectum	Onset of symptoms to operation (years)	Operation to diagnosis of carcinoma (years)	Result
Dennis & Karlson (1952)	41	2	8 8	4 5	Dead Alive
Griffen et al. (1963)	46	2			Dead Dead
Sprechler & Baden (1971)	48	1			Dead
Adson (1972)	35	2		10 17	Dead
Yudin (1973)	55	1			Dead
Gruner et al. (1975)	57	3	7 14 10	7 4 4	Dead Dead Alive
Baker et al. (1978)	374	22	1–23	3–19	13 Dead 9 Alive
*7 Other reports	256	Nil			
Total	912	33 (3·6%)			

*[Veidenheimer *et al.* (1970), Ribet *et al.* (1973), Vink & Beerstecker (1973), Mignon *et al.* (1974), Smith *et al.* (1974), Jones (1980) and Khubchandeni *et al.* (1979) report a total of 256 ileorectal anastomoses with no carcinoma recti detected]

                    Peter F. Jones

work, and would not, with more experience, have considered suitable for ileo-rectal anastomosis.

(2) No case of carcinoma of the rectal stump arose in less than 10 years from the onset of symptoms and 8 of the 22 arose more than 20 years after onset. The cumulative risk of developing a carcinoma in the rectal stump is nil at 10 years from onset, about 6% at 20 years, 9% at 25 years and 15% at 30 years.

(3) Of the 22 patients, 21 had total colonic involvement at the time of operation.

(4) If the incidence of these cases of rectal carcinoma is related to age at the onset of disease, there is no evidence that an earlier age of onset is related to a higher incidence of carcinomatous change.

(5) The importance of regular sigmoidoscopic follow-up examination is strongly emphasised by this survey and it must always be accompanied by one or more biopsies of the rectal mucosa. No conclusion is reached by the authors about the significance of dysplastic change in the mucosa, but it must always be taken as a very serious warning. However, a carcinoma can arise in ulcerative colitis without preceding dysplastic change, so this is not a consistent warning sign (Cook and Goligher, 1975).

It is difficult to place this serious complication in correct perspective but Table 21.8 shows that only 3·6% of over 900 patients followed over long periods have so far developed a reported carcinoma.

A number of these cases come from Aylett's series and we know he was prepared to use severely diseased rectums. It is not yet possible to say whether the incidence of carcinoma may be lower in rectums which appeared nearly normal at the time of anastomosis.

Crohn's disease

When Crohn's disease affects the large intestine it commonly produces severe changes around the anal canal, including strictures, fissures and fistulae, and these will generally mean that excision of the rectum must be performed if the patient is to be made comfortable. There is very little evidence that total colectomy and ileostomy with preservation of the rectum will lead to healing of the anal region, which would allow a second stage ileo-rectal anastomosis.

However, Crohn's colitis is characteristically patchy in its distribution and some patients have an almost normal rectum and anal canal even when there is severe deformity, ulceration and even fistulation in the colon. In such patients, ileo-rectal anastomosis is well worth considering.

Two of our best long-term results have been in patients with Crohn's colitis and so far only one out of our 8 patients has required rectal excision: however, this patient illustrates the progressive nature of the disease because, after developing severe peri-anal sepsis requiring rectal excision, he went on to develop recurrences throughout the small intestine from which he died.

There are only a few reports of the results of ileo-rectal anastomosis in Crohn's colitis, of which the most extensive is that of Lefton *et al.* (1975) who report 66 patients treated at the Cleveland Clinic. They were careful to limit the operation to patients with a normal or mildly inflamed rectum and they had no anastomotic leaks (but half the patients had a covering ileostomy). With an average follow-up period of 6 years, Lefton *et al.* were able to report 'excellent' results in 26 and 'satisfactory' results in 12 patients. Among the 21 unsatisfactory results, 17 patients had to have conversion to an ileostomy, mostly with rectal excision, and 4 needed revision of the ileo-rectal anastomosis. Finally, 7 patients with a loop ileostomy above the ileo-rectal anastomosis had never had the ileostomy closed. Overall, 60% of these patients secured a reasonable result, and this figure rose to 75% among those between 10 and 20 years of age. Alexander-Williams *et al.* (1974) report similar results from Birmingham, 18 of 41 patients having an excellent result and 21 being free of recurrence. Baker (1971), reporting from St. Mark's Hospital, and Weterman and Peña (1976) from Leiden, had less success with the operation. However, all are agreed that those of their patients who have secured a good result are impressively well and asymptomatic, and for this reason it is worthwhile to continue to offer ileo-rectal anastomosis to suitable patients even if a proportion (which may be as high as one-half) have to undergo later excision of the rectum.

Children and adolescents

There is a considerable amount of evidence that children and adolescents who receive an ileo-rectal anastomosis do particularly well and our own experience has confirmed this. All our surviving patients who were operated on during their school years have had an excellent result. We have had to operate and perform total colectomy on 19 children up to 17 years of age and whilst 7 needed a proctocolectomy, it was possible to perform an ileo-rectal anastomosis in 12. Only one of the 12 has required rectal excision, so a bias towards anastomosis seems to be justified.

These good results are very welcome because there are particularly strong social and emotional reasons for trying to avoid an ileostomy in young people, and it is a great deal easier to commend the idea of operation to patients and their parents when permanent ileostomy is not a part of the procedure. This is a matter of great practical importance in children and adolescents because among the serious effects of colitis in the young are retardation of growth and poor educational progress due to frequent absences from school. Total colectomy may be the only way for a child to recover health but the threat of ileostomy deters both parents and paediatricians from accepting the surgery which is really needed. Table 21.9 shows that total colectomy and ileo-rectal anastomosis can give good long-term results in about three-quarters of young patients: furthermore, if, after some years, rectal excision becomes necessary, the time during which the growing child or adolescent has not been troubled with an ileostomy may have been of great importance during the formation of friendships, undertaking apprenticeships, going to university or coming to engagement and marriage. Late excision is not necessarily to be regarded as a failure of ileo-rectal anastomosis (Jones *et al.*, 1978).

Table 21.9. *Ileo-rectal anastomosis: late results (ulcerative colitis only)*

	Total	Rectal Excision		'Good' result	
		No.	%	No.	%
All age groups					
Baker *et al.* (1978)	384	41	11		(83%)
Watts & Hughes (1977)	66	12	18	34	52
Gruner *et al.* (1975)	57	23	40	15	26
Vink & Beerstecker (1973)	50	3	6	27	54
Mignon *et al.* (1974)	48	17	35	22	45
Sprechler & Baden (1971)	48	4	8	27	56
Griffen *et al.* (1963)	47	3	7	25	53
Jones (1980	37	4	10	25	67
Adson *et al.* (1972)	35	7	20	11	31
Children only					
Aylett (1976)	28	3	10	23	82
Ehrenpreis (1966)	19	2	10	17	89
Jones (1980)	11	1	9	7	63
Nixon (1974)	10	1	10	9	90

It is also important to note the finding, already referred to, of Baker *et al.* (1978) that 'there is little evidence in the series to suggest that rectal carcinoma . . . is related to the age of onset of colitis'. This is an important finding in this large series because previous writers, such as Devroede *et al.* (1971) have suggested that onset of colitis in childhood increases the risk of carcinoma in the rectal stump. It is also worth remembering that young patients with a short history are at little or no risk of carcinoma for 10 years, and during this period ileo-rectal anastomosis may serve these patients very well.

Conclusions

The extent to which surgeons have employed ileo-rectal anastomosis has varied remarkably (Table 21.10). Aylett (1974) was prepared to use it in 96% of his large series of patients, but the surgeons at the Mayo Clinic (Adson *et al.*, 1972) and Lahey Clinic (Veidenheimer *et al.*, 1970) felt able to join the ileum to the rectum in only 10% of their patients. Those who most use this anastomosis protect the anastomosis by a proximal loop ileostomy whilst the diseased rectum heals (Aylett, 1974; Ribet *et al.*, 1973). Those who confine ileo-rectal anastomosis to patients with near-normal rectums do not need such protection and their leakage rate and consequently their mortality rate is low (Jones *et al.*, 1977) and they employ this method in one-third to one-half of their patients (Table 21.10).

Just as the degree to which ileo-rectal anastomosis is used varies widely from one surgeon to another, so do the late results (Table 21.9) and there is no common factor which explains why some surgeons have better results than others, except that children and adolescents do better than older patients. However, a majority of the surgeons reporting have obtained good long-term results in one-half to two-thirds of their patients and it is the striking good health and normal life and work of these patients which encourage continued use of the operation, especially in young people. Stool frequency is surprisingly variable but rarely more than 6 per day, and the great majority of patients say that this causes them no difficulty.

However, late relapse is a problem, although a fairly small one, but it can present suddenly with an acutely ill patient as in two of our patients. In Crohn's colitis a late recurrence is a real possibility, either in the rectum or in the ileum, but the high quality of life enjoyed by

Table 21.10. *Proportion of patients undergoing total colectomy for colitis who have an ileorectal anastomosis*

		Total Colectomies	IRA	IRA %
Ribet *et al.* (1973)	Lille	76	76	100
Aylett (1974)	Gordon Hospital	461	436	94
Vink & Beerstecker (1973)	Leyden	73	42	60
Jones (1980)	Aberdeen	112	45	40
Ehrenpreis (1966)	Stockholm (<19 y)	45	19	42
Spreckler & Baden (1971)	Copenhagen	127	48	38
Yudin *et al.* (1973)	Moscow	167	55	33
Muir (1959)	London	60	19	32
Hughes and Russell (1967)	Melbourne	234	63	27
Mignon *et al.* (1974)	Paris	250	28	11
Adson *et al.* (1972)	Mayo Clinic	350	35	10
Veidenheimer *et al.* (1970)	Lahey Clinic	387	36	9·3

the 50–60% of patients who do not suffer recurrence makes the operation well worth trying, and experience suggests that the risk of carcinoma is very low.

In conclusion, it seems right to summarise personal experience of the operation. One retains a strong impression of a number of patients who lead a virtually normal life, and this is regularly reinforced by their annual return to the follow-up clinic. On the other hand, the possibility of a carcinoma arising in the retained rectum is a risk for the patients with ulcerative colitis and a careful annual sigmoidoscopy, with several rectal biopsies, is an essential precaution to which the patient must give true informed consent before the operation is undertaken. The possibility of carcinoma arising in the retained rectal mucosa considerably enhances the attractions of operations which remove this mucosa but retain the anal canal. However, the results of ileo-anal anastomosis are currently sufficiently uncertain to make this a doubtful alternative and the interesting variant of this operation described by Parks and Nicholls (1978) will need further evaluation before it can be generally adopted. The accumulated experience of the last twenty years certainly justifies continued use of ileo-rectal anastomosis in suitable patients with Crohn's colitis, and we shall continue to use it, on a strictly selective basis, for patients with ulcerative colitis. The situation is well summed up by Baker and his colleagues (1978) when they write — 'every clinician who contemplates advising colectomy and ileo-rectal anastomosis for ulcerative colitis must form his own judgement on the benefits and risks of this type of treatment'.

ACKNOWLEDGEMENT

I am very much indebted to Dr S. W. B. Ewen for his expert advice on the histopathology of the biopsy specimens.

References

Adson M.A., Cooperman A.M. and Farrow G.M. (1972) *Arch. Surg.* **104**, 424.
Alexander-Williams J. *et al.* (1974) *Arch. Mal. App. Dig.* **63**, 588.
Aylett S.O. (1974) *Arch. Mal. App. Dig.* **63**, 585.
Aylett S.O. (1976). In *A Surgical Diversion,* ed. Clarke T.K. Squibb, London, pp. 16–26.
Baker W.N.W. (1971) *Gut,* **12**, 427.
Baker W.N.W. *et al.* (1978) *Brit. J. Surg.* **65**, 862.
Cook M.G. and Goligher J.C. (1975) *Gastroenterology,* **68**, 1127.
Dennis C. and Karlson K.E. (1952) *Surgery,* **32**, 892.
Devroede G.J. *et al.* (1971) *New Engl. J. Med.* **285**, 17.
Ehrenpreis T. (1966) *Arch. Dis. Childh.* **41**, 137.
Griffen W.O., Lillehei R.C. and Wangensteen O.H. (1963) *Surgery,* **53**, 705.
Grüner O.P.N. *et al.* (1975) *Scand. J. Gastroenterol.* **10**, Suppl. 34, 36.
Hughes E.S.R. and Russell I.S. (1967) *Dis. Colon. Rectum,* **10**, 35.
Hughes E.S.R. and Bennett R.C. (1972) *Aust. N.Z. J. Surg.* **42**, 26.
Jones P.F. (1980) Personal series reported in the present chapter.
Jones P.F., Munro A. and Ewen S.W.B. (1977) *Brit. J. Surg.* **64**, 615.
Jones P.F., Bevan P.G. and Hawley P.R. (1978) *Brit. med. J.* i, 1459.

Khubchandani I.T. *et al.* (1978) *Amer. J. Surg.* **135**, 751.
Kock N.G. (1969) *Arch. Surg.* **99**, 223.
Lefton H.B., Farmer R.G. and Fazio V. (1975) *Gastroenterology,* **69**, 612.
Lilienthal H. (1901) *Amer. Med.* **1**, 164.
Mignon M., Bonneford A. and Vilotte J. (1974) *Arch. Mal. App. Dig.* **63**, 541.
Muir E.G. (1959) *Proc. roy. Soc. Med.* **52**, Suppl. 25–27.
Munro A. and Jones P.F. (1978) *Brit. J. Surg.* **65**, 123.
Nixon H.H. (1974) *Arch. Mal. App. Dig.* **63**, 590.
Parks A.G. and Nicholls R.J. (1978) *Brit. med. J.* **ii**, 85.
Ravitch M.M. and Handelsman J.C. (1951) *Bull. Johns Hopkins Hosp.* **88**, 59.
Ribet M. *et al.* (1973) *Chirurgie,* **99**, 474.
Smith D.L., Goldman H.S. and Foote R.F. (1974) *Dis. Colon Rectum,* **17**, 681.
Sprechler M. and Baden H. (1971) *Brit. med. J.* **ii**, 527.
Veidenheimer M.C., Dailey T.H. and Meissner W.A. (1970) *Amer. J. Surg.* **119**, 375.
Vink M. and Beerstecker H.J.P. (1973) *Arch. Chir. Neerl.* **25**, 107.
Watts J.Mck. and Hughes E.S.R. (1977) *Brit. J. Surg.* **64**, 77.
Webster C.U. and Howard R.R.S. (1973) *Brit. J. Surg.* **60**, 42.
Weterman I.T. and Peña A.S. (1976) *Scand J. Gastroenterol.* **11**, 185.
Yudin I.Y. (1973) *Amer. J. Proctol.* **24**, 403.

Miscellaneous Topics

Chapter 22
Antibiotic-associated pseudomembranous colitis

M. R. B. KEIGHLEY

Pseudomembranous colitis was first described by Finney (1893). Initial reports were based entirely on autopsy material and few cases were diagnosed before death. Many early cases were recorded after surgical operations (Penner and Druckerman, 1948). The operations most frequently associated with pseudomembranous colitis were for patients with obstructive colo-rectal carcinoma (Pettet *et al.*, 1954). Early reports of this disorder were before the use of antibiotics and the disease was thought to be due to obstruction or ischaemia. More recently, pseudomembranous colitis has become regarded as a specific complication of antimicrobials. The term antibiotic–associated colitis (AAC) has been used to differentiate this relatively common disorder with a known aetiology from the disease with an identical histological appearance which was described in the pre-antibiotic era.

Reports of colitis occurring after administration of lincomycin or clindamycin implied that this might be a specific complication of this group of antimicrobials (Scott *et al.*, 1973; Viteri *et al.*, 1974). However, this disorder is now recognised to be associated with many other antimicrobials including ampicillin (Keating *et al.*, 1974; Simla *et al.*, 1976), cephazolin (Fee *et al.*, 1977), cotrimoxazole (Cameron and Thomas, 1977) and combinations of drugs, particularly the aminoglycosides with metronidazole (Kappas *et al.*, 1978).

Clinical presentation

We have reported 66 patients with AAC between March 1975 and February 1979 (Mogg *et al.*, 1979b). Twenty-three patients were males and the mean age was 59 years. The underlying disease requiring admission to hospital is listed in Table 22.1. The majority of the patients (85%) developed antibiotic—associated colitis after an operation and in 37 (56%) the operation was for disorders of the colon or rectum. The majority of these patients had a neoplasm, either of the colon (22), stomach (2), breast (1), or leukaemia (1).

The principal clinical presentation was diarrhoea which was present in all except 2 patients. The diarrhoea was usually watery but not offensive and contained excess mucus. However, it was never associated with bleeding. Only 5 patients developed severe colicky abdominal pain and 3 of these subsequently had radiological evidence of megacolon.

Fever was the other striking clinical feature which was recorded in 67% of patients. The volume and frequency of diarrhoea was variable, but frequently necessitated parenteral fluid replacement. In none of the patients was the attack of colitis associated with bleeding or perforation of the colon.

The principal laboratory findings were a leucocytosis greater than 15.0×10^6/litre in 41% of patients and a serum albumin less than 3.0 g/litre in 76%. In 24% the serum albumin fell to less than 2.5 g/litre. The mean level of serum orosomucoids was 2.7 g/litre.

Radiological features of AAC include evidence of toxic dilation on plain X-ray which was observed in only 3 of our patients. Contrast studies and colonoscopy were rarely performed because of the fear of large bowel perforation (Kappas *et al.*, 1976). However, in 8 patients having a barium enema, total colonic involvement was observed in 5

Table 22.1. *Underlying disorder in 66 patients with AAC*

Carcinoma of colon	10	(obstruction: 3)
Carcinoma of rectum	12	
Diverticular disease	4	
Rectal prolapse	11	
Small bowel obstruction	5	
Crohn's disease	1	
Gastric carcinoma	2	
Gastric ulcer	2	
Biliary disease	5	
Other	14	

cases, whilst in the remainder the mucosal abnormality was confined to the left colon.

Antimicrobials

All patients in this series had received an antibiotic prior to the onset of symptoms. A large variety of antibiotics had been prescribed and many were used in combination. The antibiotics prescribed reflect the type of operations performed. The principal antibiotics used for colo-rectal operations were the aminoglycosides with metronidazole or clindamycin, and these were the most frequent combinations associated with the disorder. Apart from lincomycin and clindamycin, the only other antimicrobials used alone and complicated by AAC were amoxy-cillin, ampicillin, cephazolin, cefuroxine, cotrimoxazole and tetracycline.

Diagnosis

The diagnosis of AAC may be difficult. The principal methods of identifying the disorder are by sigmoidoscopic appearances, rectal or colonic biopsy and, more recently, by the demonstration of a toxin in the faeces. The typical sigmoidoscopic appearances are of multiple white plaques adherent to the mucosa (Fig. 22.1). The intervening mucosa is normal and there is no blood or purulent material within the lumen. However, adequate visualisation of the mucosa may be difficult if there is profuse diarrhoea, and interpretation may be con-fused if a recent anastomosis has been performed in the rectum.

The histological appearance of antibiotic colitis is difficult to differentiate from ischaemic colitis (Price and Davies, 1977). The principal features are inflammatory changes with fibrin and polymorphs splaying out from the lamina propria, disrupted glands distended with mucin, and polymorphs covered with a pseudomembrane of epithelial debris, fribrin, mucus and polymorphs (Fig. 22.2). These appearances are readily seen if the biopsy includes a macroscopic plaque of pseudo-membrane, but is extremely unusual if the biopsy is either taken at random or is from an uninvolved segment of mucosa.

The most important advance both in our understanding of the disease and as a means of diagnosis is the observation that a faecal toxin is usually present in antibiotic—associated colitis (Larson *et al.*, 1977;

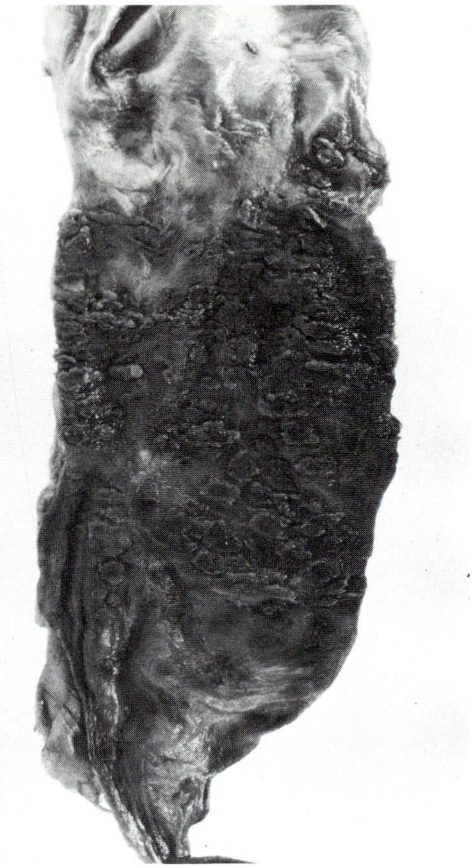

Fig. 22.1. *Macroscopic appearances of AAC.*

Rifkin *et al.*, 1977; Bartlett *et al.*, 1978; George *et al.*, 1978). The faecal toxin can be identified within 24 hours of incubating serial dilutions of faecal suspensions on monolayers of Hela cells (Fig. 22.3), embryonic lung fibroblasts or rhesus monkey kidney cells. The principal diagnostic feature is rounding and disruption of cells; these appearances are completely neutralised by incubation for 24 hours with *Clostridium sordelli* antitoxin.

In 25 patients seen in this hospital before the assay of the faecal toxin became established in August, 1977, 9 were diagnosed by sigmoidoscopy and rectal biopsy, 7 were diagnosed by histology alone and in 9 the diagnosis was only made at autopsy (Table 22.2). The reason for the

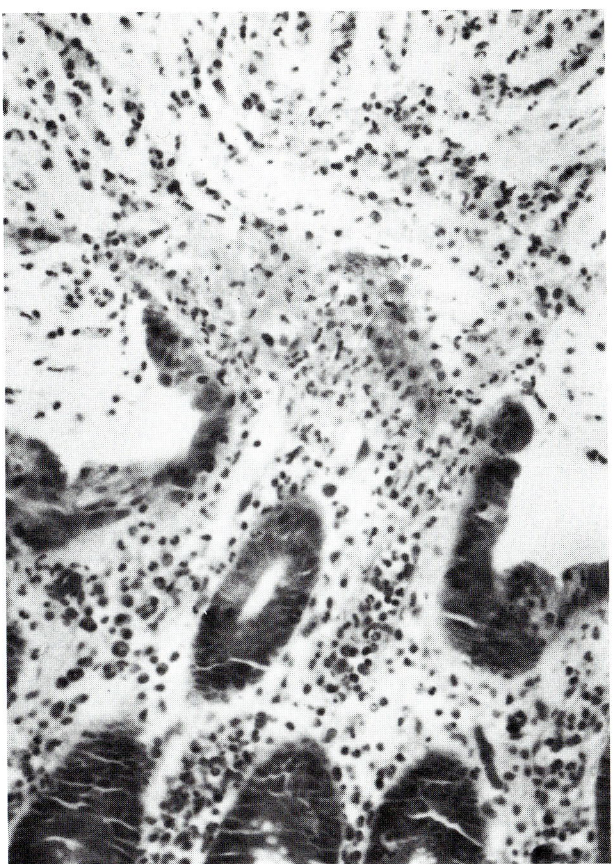

Fig. 22.2. *Histological appearances of AAC.*

high mortality in these early years was due to our failure to recognise the disorder. Six cases were mis-diagnosed as having severe sepsis (3 cases) or dehiscence of a rectal anastomosis (3 cases) and in the latter the surgeons had felt that sigmoidoscopy might be dangerous. One patient was readmitted 5 weeks after operation due to electrolyte depletion and the diagnosis was not even considered. In two cases, the diagnosis was considered but biopsy showed only non-specific changes; in both of these patients, biopsies were from a colostomy following excision of the rectum. It would appear, therefore, that biopsy is unreliable through a stoma and that rectal sparing may also be a feature of this disease.

                    M. R. B. Keighley

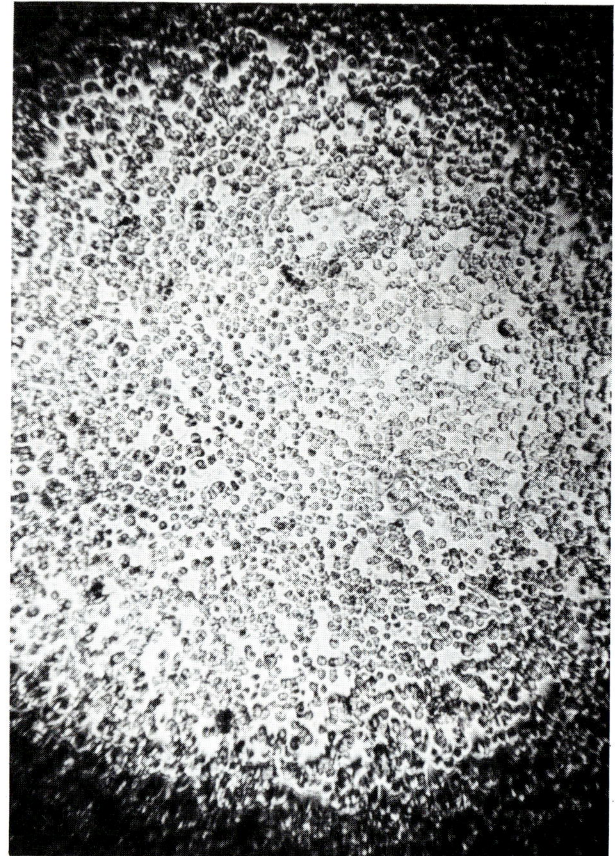

Fig. 22.3. *Toxin demonstrated on a monolayer of Hela cells.*

With the availability of a toxin assay, misdiagnosis has been reduced, since all patients with persistent diarrhoea were investigated by this means. Of the 41 patients seen since this policy was instigated in September, 1977, in only 2 was the diagnosis made at autopsy. In 11 patients, the diagnosis was established by demonstration of the toxin alone, in 21 cases the toxin findings were supported by sigmoidoscopy or histology, but in 7 patients the toxin was negative despite positive histology and biopsy. The last group probably reflect patients who were improving, since evidence of toxin may be transient even in a small number of untreated patients.

Table 22.2. *Method of diagnosis in the 66 patients with AAC*

Before availability of toxin:	
Sigmoidoscopy and histology	9
Histology alone	7
Post mortem	9
After availability of toxin:	
Sigmoidoscopy, histology and toxin	13
Sigmoidoscopy and histology only	7
Histology and toxin only	8
Toxin alone	11
Post mortem	2

Aetiology

The report that AAC was associated with a faecal toxin which could be neutralised by a clostridial antitoxin was the single most important finding to substantiate an aetiology for the disorder. An intensive search was made on both sides of the Atlantic for an organism which was capable of producing the toxin. *Clostridium sordellii* was not isolated from the faeces of patients with AAC. Independent observations from our unit and from Boston, published within 10 days of each other, reported that a different organism, *Clostridium difficile,* was present in all patients with evidence of the faecal toxin (George *et al.*, 1978; Bartlett *et al.*, 1978). Furthermore, the organism was capable of producing in broth culture a toxin which could also be neutralised by *Cl. sordellii* antitoxin and which was therefore the same as the faecal toxin. Similar observations have also been made in a hamster model pretreated with clindamycin and inoculated with *Cl. difficile* (Tedesco *et al.*, 1978). Further evidence for the disease being caused by the toxin of *Cl. difficile* has been substantiated by the rapid clinical improvement reported when treatment effectively eliminates the toxin from the colon.

It has not been established whether AAC is caused by overgrowth of *Cl. difficile,* which is normally present in very small numbers in the colon, as in staphylococcal enterocolitis. Another hypothesis is that

AAC may represent a true infection which can be transmitted from patients with the disease or chronic carriers of the organism. It is for this reason that we have recently undertaken a study to investigate the epidemiology of AAC (Mogg *et al.*, 1979a). To determine whether the disease was caused by overgrowth of a normal intestinal organism, all patients admitted to a single surgical ward were screened for *Cl. difficile* in the stool in 2 four-week periods. Of 109 patients studied, only 3 were found to carry *Cl. difficile* on admission. All three were patients who were being readmitted for a second surgical procedure and who had developed AAC during their previous admission to hospital. Although *Cl. difficile* could not be demonstrated as a normal faecal organism, a chronic carrier state was identified in patients who had had a previous attack. For this reason, the members of the nursing, medical and ward staff were screened, but in none was *Cl. difficile* isolated from the stool. It may be that the selective medium used for identifying *Cl. difficile* is incapable of detecting the organism if it is normally present in small numbers. There is circumstantial evidence that alteration of the normal faecal flora is responsible for antibiotic-associated colitis, since only 1 out of 46 patients developed AAC after receiving systemic antibiotics which had no influence on colonic flora. By contrast, 6 of 47 patients given oral agents which had a profound influence on colonic microflora developed AAC (Keighley *et al.*, 1979).

The possibility that AAC could be due to a transmissible infection was also investigated. Extensive sampling from the ward environment, the sigmoidoscopes and the lavatories failed to demonstrate *Cl. difficile* except in one instance from a bed-pan rack. The effect of moving patients to three wards which had never before been associated with AAC was also studied (Fig. 22.4). Five new cases of AAC were recorded within one month of moving a single convalescent patient to the new ward. These results suggest that cross infection had been occurring from asymptomatic carriers. As a result of sterilising the ward sigmoidoscopes and effective treatment of all asymptomatic carriers by eliminating *Cl. difficile* from their stools, AAC has been almost completely abolished in our surgical unit.

Incidence

In order to try to determine the incidence of AAC, a prospective study was undertaken of all patients admitted to our unit from 1st September

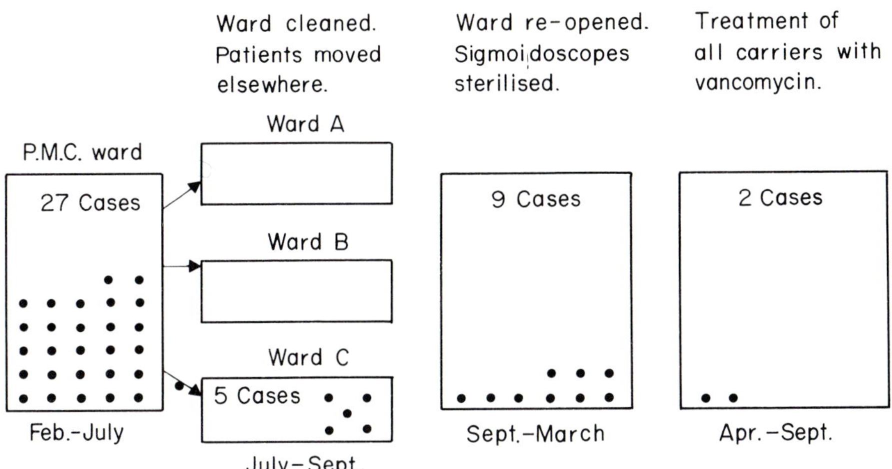

Fig. 22.4. *Epidemiological study.*

1977 to 28th April 1978. Every patient with post-operative diarrhoea, defined as more than three stools a day or colostomy output greater than 1 litre per 24 hours, was studied for evidence of toxins or *Cl. difficile* in the stool (Keighley *et al.*, 1978a). Of the 241 patients admitted for major intestinal operations, 119 (50%) had received antibiotics and 58 (24%) had diarrhoea. Of the group with diarrhoea, 9 had a neutralisable faecal toxin and in all of them toxigenic *Cl. difficile* was also isolated. This represents a 4% incidence of AAC in patients undergoing gastro-intestinal operations. The study also showed that diarrhoea was significantly more common ($p < 0.002$) in patients exposed to antibiotics (39%), than in patients who had received no antibiotics (10%).

Antibacterial sensitivity of *Cl. difficile*

The sensitivity of *Cl. difficile* to antibacterial agents has important therapeutic implications. The results from our laboratory indicated that the sensitivity of *Cl. difficile* from patients with AAC differed from *Cl. difficile* isolated from other patients. Toxigenic strains of *Cl. difficile* were invariably resistant to aminoglycosides and frequently resistant to penicillin, clindamycin and tetracyline (Burdon *et al.*, 1979). All of our isolates have been sensitive to metronidazole; however, the therapeutic value of metronidazole has been questioned since it is rapidly absorbed by the small bowel so that the level of metronidazole in faecal material is very low. All our isolates of *Cl. difficile* were inhibited by 16 mg/litre of vancomycin. Vancomycin is an agent which is poorly absorbed and even small doses (125 mg four times a day) provides faecal levels of between 60 to 760 mg/litre.

Therapy

Two forms of therapy for AAC have been investigated by randomised controlled trials. The compounds which were studied included vancomycin which was thought to be capable of eradicating *Cl. difficile* from the colon and an ion-exchange resin (colestipol) which had been shown to absorb the toxin but which was unlikely to influence counts of *Cl. difficile* (Tedesco *et al.*, 1979). The trials were performed on a consecutive series of 82 patients with post-operative diarrhoea within a single surgical ward. All patients entering the trials had an initial sigmoidoscopy and biopsy. Stools were collected before treatment for detection of toxin and *Cl. difficile*. Patients were then allocated to vancomycin 125 mg six hourly (n = 22), colestipol 10 g six hourly (n = 17) or placebo vancomycin or placebo colestipol. A repeat sigmoidoscopic biopsy and stool samples for toxins and *Cl. difficile* were obtained on the last day of treatment (day 5). There were 44 patients in the vancomycin trial and 38 in the colestipol trial. Since the criteria for entry and the nature of the placebo was identical in both trials, the results of both placebo groups have been combined (n = 43). The underlying clinical conditions and prescribed antibiotics were similar in each treatment group. The patients were classified as belonging to one of three types. Type A included patients with toxin and *Cl. difficile*, Type B were patients with *Cl. difficile* alone, and Type C were patients with neither organism or toxin.

Treatment with vancomycin was associated with rapid elimination of toxin and *Cl. difficile* from the stool whereas colestipol and placebo had no influence on toxin titre or the counts of *Cl. difficile* (Table 22.3). There was also a rapid clinical response in 75% of the patients with toxin or the organism in the stool who received vancomycin (Table 22.4) as compared with a 36% and a 22% response in the colestipol and placebo group respectively.

These results have confirmed that oral vancomycin is the treatment

Table 22.3. *Bacteriological response to various types of treatment*

(a) Toxin present (Type A)

	Vancomycin	Colestipol	Placebo
Day 1	7	5	5
Day 5	1	5	6

(b) *Cl. difficile* present (Types A and B)

	Vancomycin	Colestipol	Placebo
Day 1	10	10	10
Day 5	1	11	10

of choice for AAC (Keighley *et al.*, 1978b). Furthermore, vancomycin reduces the risk of asymptomatic carriers since the organism is usually eliminated from the colon. Results of treatment with ion-exchange resins (Kreutzer *et al.*, 1979) in our experience have been disappointing, presumably because the causative toxigenic organism has not been eliminated from the stool.

Conclusions

Our observations indicate that AAC is still a potentially fatal complication of antibacterial therapy. The diagnosis of AAC by sigmoidoscopy and biopsy is not always reliable and should depend upon the demonstration of a neutralisable toxin in the stool. Successful treatment and

Table 22.4. *Clinical response to various types of treatment as judged by the number of patients with a normal bowel habit by the end of treatment*

	Vancomycin	Colestipol	Placebo
Types A and B	9/12	5/14	3/14
Type C	6/10	1/3	12/29

prevention of epidemics of AAC relies upon eliminating toxin-producing strains of *Cl. difficile* from the colon and this can be achieved with oral vancomycin.

References

Bartlett J.G., Chang T.W., Gurwith M., Gorbach S.L. and Onderdonk A.B. (1978) *New Engl. J. Med.* **298**, 531.

Burdon D.W., Brown J., Youngs D.J., Arabi Y., Shinagawa N., Alexander-Williams J., Keighley M.R.B. and George R.H. (1979) *J. Antimicrob. Chemother.* **5**, 307.

Cameron A. and Thomas M. (1977) *Brit. Med. J.* i, 1321.

Fee H.J., Ament M.E. and Holmes E.C. (1977) *Amer. J. Surg.* **133**, 247.

Finney J.M.T. (1893) *Bull. Johns Hopkins Hosp.* **4**, 53.

George R.H., Symonds J.M., Dimock F., Brown J.D., Arabi Y., Shinagawa N., Keighley M.R.B., Alexander-Williams J. and Burdon D.W. (1978) *Brit. Med. J.* i, 695.

Kappas A., Shinagawa N., Arabi Y., Thompson H., Burdon D.W., Dimock F., George R.H., Alexander-Williams J. and Keighley M.R.B. (1978) *Brit. Med. J.* i, 675.

Keating J.P., Frank A.L. and Barton L.L. (1974) *Amer. J. Dis. Childh.* **128**, 369.

Keighley M.R.B., Arabi Y., Alexander-Williams J., Youngs D. and Burdon D.W. (1979) *Lancet,* i, 894.

Keighley M.R.B., Burdon D.W., Alexander-Williams J., Shinagawa N., Arabi Y., Thompson H., Youngs D., Bentley S. and George R.H. (1978a) *Lancet,* ii, 1165.

Keighley M.R.B., Burdon D.W., Arabi Y., Alexander-Williams J., Thompson H., Youngs D., Johnson M., Bentley S., George R.H. and Mogg G.A.G. (1978b) *Brit. med. J.* i, 1667.

Kreutzer E.W. and Milligan F.D. (1978) *Johns Hopkins Hosp. Med. J.* **143**, 67.

Larson H.E., Parry J.V., Price A.B., Davies D.R., Dolby J., Tyrell D.A.J. (1977) *Brit. med. J.* i, 1246.

Mogg G.A.G., Burdon D.W., Alexander-Williams J., Youngs D., Johnson M., George R.H. and Keighley M.R.B. (1979a) *Gut,* **20**, A459.

Mogg G.A.G., Keighley M.R.B., Burdon D.W., Alexander-Williams J., Youngs D., Johnson M., Bentley S. and George R.H. (1979b) *Brit. J. Surg.* **66**, 738.

Penner A. and Druckerman L.J. (1948) *Gastroenterology,* **11**, 478.

Pettet J.D., Baggenstoss A.H.W. and Dearing W. (1954) *Surg. Gynec. Obst.* **98**, 546.

Price A.B. and Davies D.R. (1977) *J. clin. Path.* **30**, 1.

Rifkin G.D., Fekety F.R., Silva J. and Sack R.B. (1977) *Lancet,* ii, 1232.

Scott A.J., Nicholson G.I. and Kerr A.R. (1973) *Lancet,* ii, 1232.

Simla S., Kouvalainen K. and Makela P. (1976) *Lancet,* ii, 317.

Tedesco F., Markham R., Gurwith M., Christie D. and Bartlett J.G. (1978) *Lancet,* ii, 226.

Tedesco F.J., Napier J., Gamble W., Chang Te Wen and Bartlett J.G. (1979) *J. clin. Gastroenterol.* **1**, 51.

Viteri A.L., Howard P.H. and Dyck W.P. (1974) *Gastroenterology,* **66**, 1137.

Chapter 23
Ischaemic disease of the colon

ADRIAN MARSTON

The main blood supply of the intestine comes from the coeliac axis and from the superior and inferior mesenteric arteries. The proximal half of the colon is supplied by the superior mesenteric artery (SMA) and the distal half by the inferior mesenteric artery (IMA) with some contribution from the internal iliac arteries. The anatomical arrangement is variable, depending on the way in which these main arteries interconnect. There are no complicated vascular arcades such as are found in the mesentery of the small intestine but the marginal artery serves the same purpose. The viability of a segment of colon following occlusion of a major vessel largely depends on the state of this artery. It is often poorly developed or absent in the region of the splenic flexure, which is the junction between the areas supplied by the SMA and IMA. It is therefore not surprising that this part of the colon is especially prone to ischaemic damage.

The marginal artery gives off two sets of vessels, the vasa recta and vasa brevia, which penetrate alternate aspects of the bowel wall and communicate in a rich submucosal plexus, from which penetrating branches run up between the crypts to supply the mucosa. Arterio-venous anastomoses are present but little is known about their function.

There have been few quantitative studies of colonic blood flow in man and most statements about it are based on analogy with the findings in experimental animals. The relationship of blood pressure to blood flow in the intestine is not linear. Within the physiological range, the flow does not vary greatly with alterations of pressure at the origin of the main vessel although, if the pressure becomes very low, there is a sharp reduction in flow, perhaps due to the input pressure becoming less than the critical closing pressure of the intestinal arterioles. The distal blood flow is influenced by the position and diameter of the part of the bowel concerned. For example, a kinked or distended loop has a diminished blood supply. This may be the reason why the intestinal changes are often patchy and the extent of the necrosis variable following a major vascular occlusion.

Principal causes of colonic ischaemia

Surgical interruption of the blood supply

Radiological injury

Spontaneous thrombosis of the colonic vessels

Small vessel disease

Low flow states

Obstruction

Venous disease

Infarction of unknown origin

Surgical interruption of the blood-supply

With the development of radical surgery for cancer of the colon, surgeons began to employ high ligation of the arterial trunks to facilitate wide lymphatic clearance. However, Goligher (1954) described a 25% incidence of devitalization of the terminal colon following high ligation of the IMA. It is questionable whether high ligation has any effect on the prognosis of colonic cancer and, in view of the risk of producing ischaemic damage, this procedure should probably be abandoned.

In the early 1950s, surgeons began to treat abdominal aneurysms by reconstructing the lower aorta. This frequently involved sacrificing one or more of its visceral branches, in particular the inferior mesenteric artery. Cannon (1955) reported a patient who died from unsuspected gangrene of the left colon ten days after an emergency operation for aneurysm. Smith and Szilagyi (1960) described twelve cases of ischaemia of the descending colon in 120 aortic resections. The whole question of colonic damage following aortic reconstruction has been reviewed by Johnson and Nasbeth (1974), who found an overall incidence of 99 cases in 6,100 patients (1·5%).

Radiological injury

The colon may occasionally show evidence of damage after abdominal angiography, but it is uncertain from the published reports whether the contrast medium or the trauma of cannulation is to blame. Experimental work suggests that the gut is very tolerant of concentrated angiographic media (Killen *et al.*, 1967). The newer media are probably much less toxic than those formerly in use.

Spontaneous thrombosis of the colonic vessels

As in the small intestine, mucosal damage may result from any condition in which there is inflammation of small arteries, such as polyarteritis nodosa, systemic lupus erythematosus, dermatomyositis, Wegener's granuloma and anaphylactoid purpura. The colon may suffer radiation damage, for example when radiotherapy is employed to treat uterine cancer, and this damage largely results from the effects of radiation on the small blood vessels.

Low-flow states

In a low-flow state, such as may occur in cardiac failure or severe shock, the blood supply may fail. The resulting inflammatory damage is more rapid and more harmful than a similar process in the small intestine due to the presence of large numbers of pathogenic bacteria. Of particular importance are the clostridia, which are present in the colons of one in every three healthy human subjects.

Obstruction

Blood-flow in the wall of the intestine is dependent on intraluminal pressure, radial muscle tension and diameter, quite apart from vascular influence. The characteristic radiological and pathological changes of ischaemic colitis occur frequently in the segment of bowel immediately proximal to an obstructing carcinoma (the so-called 'stercoral' ulceration)

(Boley and Schwartz, 1971; Herrmann *et al.*, 1965). Sometimes, in fact, the clinical effects of the ischaemic lesion may be sufficiently severe as to mask the presence of the tumor. Other factors leading to obstruction of the lumen of the large bowel, such as prolapse, volvulus, adhesions or narrowing of the site of a colostomy, may in the same way give rise to local ischaemic change.

Venous occlusion

Experimental studies have demonstrated that extensive venous thrombosis leads to a haemorrhagic type of infarction, with gross oedema (Marcuson *et al.*, 1972). As this lesion matures, it comes to resemble ever more closely the late results of arterial occlusion.

By the time X-rays can be taken and histological material becomes available, it may be impossible to decide whether the original causation of the infarct was on the arterial or the venous side.

If the ischaemia is severe and prolonged, there is progressive destruction of the colonic wall, ending in full-thickness necrosis, sloughing and rupture. At the other end of the scale, a transient episode of ischaemia may resolve completely and be followed by no histological abnormality. An intermediate state exists in which the remaining blood supply to the bowel is insufficient for the needs of the more specialised tissues, the mucosa and muscle, but at the same time enough remains to preserve overall viability. In these cases there is an initial brisk inflammatory response, which is followed by ulceration of the mucosa and gradual replacement of the muscle layers with fibrous tissue, resulting in a stricture of the bowel.

Gangrene of the colon

Clinical picture

The typical patient is middle-aged or elderly and has a background of degenerative cardiovascular disease, such as hypertension, episodes of left ventricular failure or myocardial infarction. There is usually no pre-existing history of bowel disturbance and the onset of the illness is sudden and dramatic, with severe generalised abdominal pain, which is at first colicky but rapidly becomes continuous. Almost all patients vomit early in the course of the illness, and diarrhoea is a very frequent feature, although bleeding is unusual. Over the course of the next few hours this clinical picture gives way to one of progressive abdominal distension, accompanied by thirst, restlessness, air-hunger, and all the symptoms of circulatory collapse.

Examination of the abdomen reveals the signs of a widespread peritonitis with diffuse tenderness, rigidity and absent bowel sounds. Rectal examination may reveal dark blood.

X-ray appearances

In the very early stages of the illness, the plain film of the abdomen is normal. After a few hours, the prominent feature is progressive dilatation of the large bowel and, later, of the small bowel, suggesting toxic megacolon or volvulus. A barium enema is clearly inappropriate because of the severity of the illness. The value of emergency aortography is debatable.

Laboratory findings

Early leucocytosis is the rule. There is progressive haemoconcentration with a rise in haematocrit, accompanied by metabolic acidosis with elevated blood urea and potassium. The serum enzymes follow no consistent pattern.

Management

The patient should be resuscitated and prepared for immediate emergency laparotomy. On opening the abdomen, it is immediately obvious that a length of colon has undergone ischaemic necrosis. The part involved may extend for any distance between the rectosigmoid and the caecum. It is, however, unusual to find involvement below the distal pelvic colon. The bowel is resected between non-crushing clamps, which are placed well wide of the abnormal area. The mucosa is then inspected carefully, and the clamps released, in order to confirm that there is arterial bleeding from the cut ends. Usually, the mucosal damage is considerably more extensive than would have been suspected from outside, and in this case it is necessary to cut the bowel back still further, in order to be certain of having removed all ischaemic tissue.

No attempt is made to achieve a primary anastomosis. The proximal end of the bowel is exteriorised in any convenient position on the abdominal wall, and the distal end either brought out in the same way, or closed and dropped back, according to the length and position of the bowel affected. The peritoneal cavity is then washed out with saline, and the wound closed with appropriate drainage.

Results

It is generally agreed that colonic gangrene carries a mortality of 80–90%. However, the figures are biased by the fact that the diagnosis is usually made at a late stage or even only at autopsy (Marcuson, 1972; Marston, 1972). With modern methods of resuscitation and rapid emergency surgery, there is every reason to suppose that this very high mortality can be reduced.

Ischaemic colitis

The term 'ischaemic colitis' is nowadays applied to the non-gangrenous form of the disease, which varies from a transient episode of inflammation to more severe disease which gives rise to a fibrous stricture (Marston *et al.*, 1966).

Clinical picture

This is typically a disease of the middle-aged and elderly. The onset is acute and the first symptom is generally a sharp pain in the left iliac fossa spreading across the abdomen and up into the epigastrium. This is followed by the passage of a small motion mixed with dark blood. The bleeding is quite characteristic, being moderate in amount, dark, mixed with stool and sometimes containing clots.

If examined at this stage of the disease, the patient is often not severely ill, although the temperature and pulse are raised. There is extreme tenderness in the left iliac fossa and in the pelvis, with dark blood on the fingerstall following rectal examination.

Endoscopy

Examination with the rigid sigmoidoscope does not usually bring the lesion into view as the area affected lies above the reach of the instrument. However, there are a few reports in the literature where the diagnosis has been made by this means (Carter *et al.*, 1959). The appearances described are of irregular heaped-up bluish purple mucosa, with oedema and contact bleeding. Colonoscopy is obviously going to be extremely useful in the early diagnosis of the disease. As yet, insufficient experience has accumulated, but at the same time no complications or disasters have been reported.

Laboratory studies

Laboratory studies are not of much value. There is almost invariably a polymorph leucocytosis, of 15,000 upwards, and the serum enzymes may be raised, as in colonic gangrene.

Radiology

A plain X-ray will often show an area of large bowel whose intraluminal gas shadow demonstrates 'thumb printing'. At a later stage in the disease, there may be signs of small bowel obstruction, with dilatation of the ileum and fluid levels.

The value of angiography is doubtful. While there are many reports in the literature of radiologically demonstrated arterial blocks, non-occlusive disease appears to be more frequent, so that a negative angiogram does not exclude the diagnosis. It is certainly not required as a routine examination in every case.

The barium enema is most useful (Fig. 23.1). The changes are characteristic: an abnormal segment of colon is seen, usually around the splenic flexure which is, as a rule, clearly demarcated from the adjoining bowel. This segment is always narrowed, and the narrowing varies from slight to complete obstruction. Its length varies from a few centimetres to involvement of the whole of the transverse and descending colon. The normal haustral pattern is lost and there is rigidity of the segment, as shown by screening and serial films. In detail the following features are seen. Polypoid change (called 'thumb printing') consists of rounded filling defects in the barium-filled colon. Mucosal irregularity presents either as smooth ridges, projecting into the lumen, or else as craters. Tubular narrowing is self-explanatory, and sacculation consists of smooth out-pouchings of the colonic wall. Generally speaking, polypoid change and mucosal irregularity are seen early in the course of the disease.

The two conditions with which ischaemic colitis is most frequently

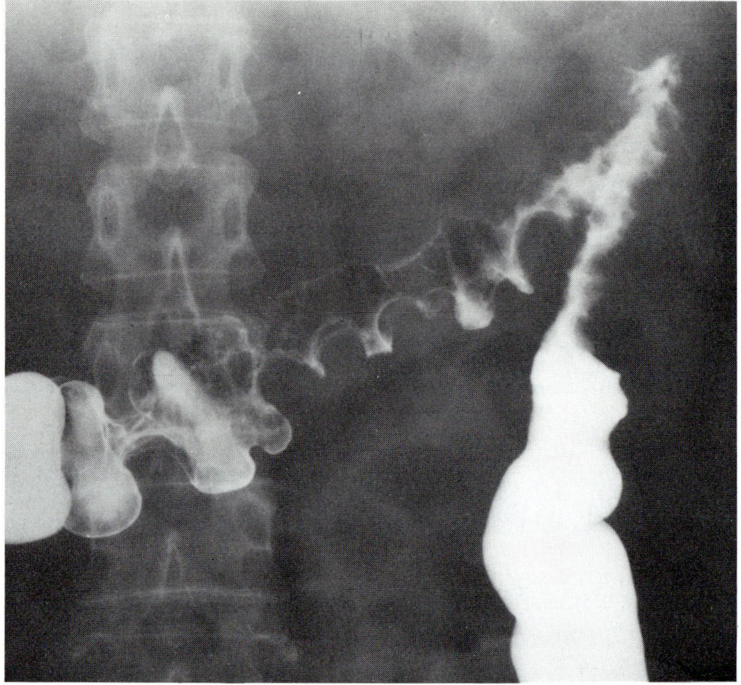

Fig. 23.1. *Ischaemic colitis affecting the colon in the region of the splenic flexure. Barium enema appearances at an early stage, showing 'thumb-printing' and loss of haustral pattern.*

confused are proctocolitis and Crohn's disease. In the later stages of the illness, particularly if a short stricture has developed, it may be difficult to distinguish this from an annular neoplasm. The main distinguishing points are the absence of the 'shouldering' and 'half-shadowing' which are so characteristic of carcinoma.

Management

Once the diagnosis has been established, treatment should in almost every case be expectant. That is to say, the patient is rested in bed, given an intravenous or enteral fluid regimen, according to the degree of peritoneal irritation, and monitored by daily leucocyte counts and haematocrit readings. It is our practice to give antibiotics (ampicillin, gentamicin, metronidazole) as it has been established that such therapy lessens the effect of colonic ischaemia in experimental animals (Benjamin *et al.*, 1960).

On this expectant regimen, there are three possible sequelae. These are:—

1. Progression to gangrene
2. Resolution (formerly described as 'transient ischaemia')
3. Formation of a stricture

Fortunately, it is extremely rare for a patient with acute non-gangrenous ischaemic colitis to develop gangrene of the colon. The usual course of events is for the symptoms to settle rapidly over the course of a few days, although they may persist for a week or two. Subsequently, a barium enema is likely to show a normal colon, or one with minimal involvement. Sometimes, probably in about 50% of all cases, a fibrous stricture develops (Fig. 23.2), but this is frequently asymptomatic and does not in itself require treatment. Strictures pronounced enough to cause obstructive symptoms should be resected.

In our series of 58 strictures, 49 patients underwent resection, of whom four died (Marcuson, 1972). Of the remaining nine patients treated conservatively, one died from a cerebrovascular accident. However, it should be borne in mind that this series includes a number of cases seen in the early 1960s, when ischaemic colitis was much less well recognised, and many of these patients would not be operated upon today.

Pathological changes

For detailed accounts of the pathological appearances the reader is referred to the writings of Morson (1972) and Allen (1971).

Differential diagnosis

In a typical case presenting as an emergency, the diagnosis should be fairly straightforward, particularly if there is associated rectal bleeding. The main conditions with which it is to be confused are:—

1. Infective gastroenteritis
2. Acute diverticular disease, including ruptured pericolic abscess, and perforation of the colon
3. Acute ulcerative colitis
4. Acute Crohn's disease of the large bowel
5. Pseudomembranous colitis

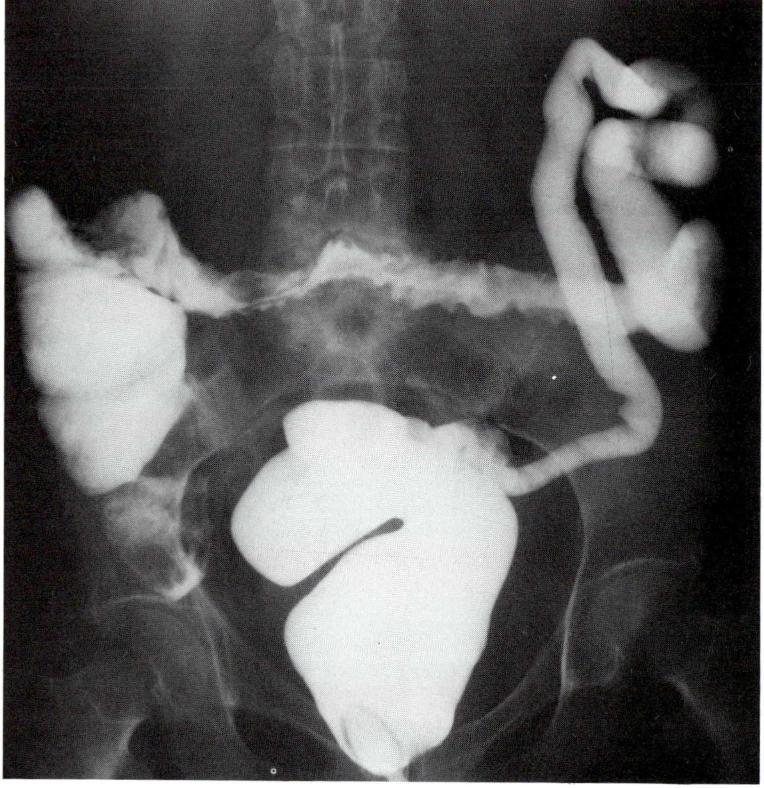

Fig. 23.2. *Ischaemic colitis. Barium enema showing a long smooth stricture of the colon which was a sequel to an attack of ulcerative colitis.*

6. Perforation of a hollow viscus, such as the stomach or duodenum, with peritonitis tracking down the left side of the abdomen
7. Acute pancreatitis
8. Left-sided renal colic
9. Leaking abdominal aortic aneurysm.

It is quite likely that many episodes of abdominal pain and diarrhoea, particularly in the older age groups, which are diagnosed as gastroenteritis or diverticular disease, may be due to transient episodes of ischaemia. There is no way to prove this point, but common sense would suggest that this is so. The main feature which distinguishes ischaemia from other conditions is the presence of the characteristic dark rectal bleeding, although this occurs only in some two-thirds of cases

(Marcuson, 1972). Often, the diagnosis is not made immediately, but comes to light only with the barium enema.

When seen later in the course of the illness, the condition may closely resemble Crohn's disease. The most important distinguishing features are the characteristic age range of the patients, the association with degenerative cardiovascular disease, and the distinctive radiological appearances.

Summary and conclusions

Ischaemic disease of the colon is now a well-recognised clinical condition, which usually occurs spontaneously but may follow surgical interference with the vasculature. Two quite distinct forms of the illness occur. In the first, there is full-thickness necrosis of the colonic wall (gangrene of the colon), which presents as an abdominal catastrophe, requires urgent excisional surgery, and carries a high mortality. The second form of the illness (ischaemic colitis) presents with acute abdominal pain associated with diarrhoea and rectal bleeding. Only a very small proportion of the cases develop gangrene. In the great majority, the symptoms settle with medical treatment over the course of a few days or a week or two. About 50% of the patients managed conservatively develop a fibrous stricture in the colon, but only a minority of these strictures give rise to obstructive symptoms and require resection.

References

Allen A.C. (1971). In *Vascular Diseases of the Intestine* ed. Boley S.J. New York, Appleton Century Crofts.
Benjamin H.B., Potos W.B., Marnocha J. and Bartenbach G.E. (1960) *J. Amer. Geriat. Soc.* **8**, 847.
Boley S.J., Schwartz S.S. (1971). In *Vascular Disorders of the Intestine*. New York, Appleton Century Crofts, p. 640.
Cannon J.A. (1955) *Amer. J. Surg.* **90**, 315.
Carter R., Vannix R., Hinshaw D.B., Stafford C.E. (1959) *Surgery*, **46**, 845.
Goligher J.C. (1954) *Brit. J. Surg.* **41**, 351.
Herrman J.W., Paine J.R., Stubbe N.J. (1965) *Surgery*, **57**, 647.
Johnson W.C., Nabseth D.C. (1974) *Ann. Surg.* **180**, 312.
Killen D.A., Sewell R., Foster J.H. (1967) *Amer. J. Surg.* **114**, 904.
Marcuson R.W., Stewart J.O., Marston A. (1972) *Gut*, **13**, 1.
Marcuson R.W. (1972) *Clinics in Gastroenterology*, **1**, 745.

 Adrian Marston

Marston A. (1972) *Ann. roy. Coll. Surg. Engl.* **50**, 29.
Marston A., Pheils M.T., Thomas M.L., Morson B.C. (1966) *Gut,* 7, 1.
Morson B.C. (1972) *Clinics in Gastroenterology,* **1**, 765.
Smith R.F. and Szilagyi D.E. (1960) *Arch. Surg.* **80**, 806.

Chapter 24
Surgical management of severe obesity

R. M. BADDELEY

Obesity is not a major hazard to life except in younger, massively overweight males below the age of 35 years (Bray, 1978). It is, however, more likely to be complicated by risk factors such as hypertension, hyperlipidaemia and diabetes, so that the mortality from cardiovascular disease is higher than that in the non-obese. The greater the obesity, the higher the mortality; at 90% above standard body weight, the excess mortality is 16 times greater than normal. Obese men, 45 kg overweight or more and 30 years of age, have a life expectancy of only 14 to 16 years (Metropolitan Life Data).

Apart from premature death, massively obese persons are prone to morbid complications, such as spondylosis, osteoarthritis, bronchitis, dyspepsia due to gallstones and hiatus hernia, cirrhosis, varicose veins and ulceration, gravitational oedema and menstrual disturbances. Psycho-social complications of obesity may result in depression or suicide. There is a greater surgical mortality and morbidity due to deep vein thrombosis and embolism, wound sepsis and chest complications.

All these hazards can be minimised by weight reduction but the results of conventional dietary measures are often unsatisfactory. Thus, in a few, it is judicious to resort to surgical measures. The latter include panniculectomy or lipectomy, dieting enforced by dental splintage, jejuno-ileal bypass and gastric bypass or plication.

Panniculectomy

This type of procedure is of limited clinical value, being mainly cosmetic. It is of psychiatric value in patients suffering from depression and loss of confidence due to their appearance. It is also appropriate in those who have masses of redundant skin as a result of marked weight reduction. Massively obese patients often suffer from back-ache, due in part to spondylosis and also to loss of normal spinal curvature caused by the pendulous abdomen. Removal of the abdominal apron may restore spinal curvature, thereby relieving the symptom.

Dental splintage

Many patients break their dietary restraint when depressed or anxious and, as a result, rapidly nullify their hard-won weight reduction. The use of mandibulo-maxillary fixation can restrain the patient at such times and strictly enforce the desired calorie reduction.

It is essential that these patients should have adequate natural dentition and preliminary dental treatment is often required. After fitting the splints, the patient is placed on an 800 K calorie fluid diet containing iron and vitamin supplements. Follow-up at monthly intervals is enforced to encourage the patient, and at 3 months it is usual to remove the splints for dental hygiene purposes.

The author has treated over 70 patients by this method. Of the first 53, 42 completed 6 months of dental splintage and achieved an average weight loss of 4·15 kg per month, or 25·8 ± 9·63 kg over the whole period (Baddeley, 1979a).

This technique is effective in those patients who adhere fully to the regimen. Clearly there is a risk of regaining weight when the restraint is removed and it is probable that the long-term results are no better than conventional dietary treatment.

Gastrointestinal techniques

Indications

The criteria for selection of patients for jejuno-ileal bypass are clearly defined. Patients must have chronic simple obesity of at least 5 years' duration which has proved refractory to properly supervised dietary measures, and which is at least 45 kg or 100% above the standard weight for age, height and sex. The patient must fully understand the radical nature of the procedure and the possibility of mortality and potential side-effects. Above all, they must agree to attend regularly for reassessment as out-patients.

Contra-indications

The contra-indications should be strictly applied. Patients who have not fulfilled the criteria already mentioned should be excluded. Patients over the age of 50 years do not tolerate well this type of surgery and those of below average intelligence should be excluded as they are not liable to follow the instructions given or to attend regularly for follow-up. Patients with primary psychiatric disturbances are unpredictable in their post-operative behaviour and should be excluded. However, those who are depressed as a result of their obesity are eminently suitable. A history of alcoholism and evidence of cirrhosis, heart disease or renal failure are strong contra-indications. The presence of other complications of obesity, such as diabetes, hypertension and osteoarthritis, are not contra-indications.

Jejuno-ileal bypass

The management of massive obesity by iatrogenic malabsorption was pioneered by Payne and DeWind (1969). They found that an end-to-side jejuno-ileal bypass, retaining 35 cm of jejunum and 10 cm of terminal ileum in intestinal continuity, evoked satisfactory and sustained weight reduction. The bypassed bowel was retained, defunctioned, but available for re-anastomosis in the event of hazardous side effects. Subsequently, there have been modifications in detail although the basic concept has been retained. Scott *et al.* (1971) claimed that end-to-end anastomosis gave more consistent weight loss but it is now established that there is no significant difference between the two techniques (Baddeley, 1979b). Variation in the lengths of jejunum and ileum used makes little difference as long as the total length of small bowel in continuity is not more than 50 cm. Popular dimensions now used are 30 cm of jejunum anastomosed to the terminal 20 cm of ileum (Scott *et al.*, 1977).

More recently, Hallburg and Holmgren (1978) have further modified jejuno-ileal bypass by additional anastomosis of the upper excluded end of the jejunum to the gallbladder. This technique facilitates absorption of bile salts in the ileum, thereby reducing the problem of diarrhoea which inevitably occurs during the early weeks after the operation. Scopinaro *et al.* (1979) have devised a technique of bilio-pancreatic bypass but the long-term results remain to be evaluated.

Post-operative care

A high-protein, low-carbohydrate, low-fat diet of 1200—1500 K calories
is advised as soon as alimentation is re-established. Fluid intake is
limited to 1·5 litres daily to minimise diarrhoea, for which an anti-
diarrhoeal and potassium supplement are also prescribed. Each patient
is seen regularly after discharge home for full blood count, serum
electrolyte estimations, liver function test and estimation of serum
vitamin B_{12}, folate, iron and iron binding capacity. Whole body
potassium estimation and percutaneous liver biopsy and bone biopsy
may be indicated from time to time.

Beneficial effects of jejuno-ileal bypass

These are: significant weight loss which is sustained over the long term,
good psycho-social rehabilitation, improved glucose tolerance, reduction
of fasting serum lipids, cholesterol and triglyceride values. Improved
respiratory function occurs in most patients and reduction of hypertension in many.

WEIGHT REDUCTION

This is most marked during the first year when an average of 32% of
the original body weight is lost. Further gradual reduction occurs over
the next 6—12 months but by 2 years it ceases altogether. An average
overall loss of about 36% of original body weight has been reported by
most authors (Baddeley, 1979a and b). Weight regain of 7—10 kg may
occur thereafter but is easily controlled by sensible dietary restraint.
Weight loss of one-third of the original weight may still leave a patient
considerably above the standard body weight; further reduction can be
achieved by carefully supervised dieting or dieting enforced by dental
splintage. Further shortening of the jejunum or ileum is not recommended nor is conversion of end-to-side to end-to-end anastomosis
or *vice-versa*.

PSYCHO-SOCIAL REHABILITATION

This is very gratifying in massively obese persons, especially women,
who are prone to secondary depression and social limitation as a result
of loss of self-esteem, fear of rejection and distortion of body image.

The benefits of weight reduction are seen as an early euphoria followed by self-confidence, assertiveness, and physical and social activity. Eating habits become more conventional and compulsive hyperphagia is reduced. Marital relationships are often improved as are the chances of employment and economic rehabilitation. A few patients, however, exhibit undesirable side-effects, which include depression, over-assertiveness and promiscuity. Patients suffering from endogenous depression may be made worse and thus the importance of careful psychiatric assessment in case selection for this type of surgery cannot be over-emphasised.

IMPROVED GLUCOSE TOLERANCE

Obesity and diabetes are frequently associated and can be rectified by weight reduction. This was well illustrated by the report of Fielding and Baddeley (1978) who found normal fasting blood glucose values in 12 out of 13 diabetics 9—44 months after jejuno-ileal bypass. In 8 patients glucose tolerance tests reverted to normal, 4 improved but were still mildly abnormal, and one retained a florid diabetic type curve. None of the patients subsequently required hypoglycaemic therapy. This beneficial change is related to weight loss rather than to impaired carbohydrate absorption.

REDUCTION IN FASTING LIPID VALUES

This is usually dramatic. Serum cholesterol levels fall by 40—45% within 3 months (DeWind and Payne, 1976; Scott *et al.*, 1977). This reduction is sustained for 5 years and more (Baddeley, 1979b). Serum triglyceride values show similar trends and lipoprotein electrophoretic patterns often return to normal.

These changes result from interruption of the enterohepatic circulation of bile salts and from fatty acid malabsorption resulting from the small amount of ileum available for absorption.

Mortality and morbidity

The operative mortality varies from 0—6% due largely to pulmonary embolism, myocardial infarction and, to a lesser extent, sepsis, wound dehiscence and peritonitis. Overall mortality averages 3·1% (Bray *et al.*, 1977), ranging from 0—11·5%. The main cause of death is hepatic failure; less frequently, myocardial infarction, pulmonary embolism, intestinal obstruction and, rarely, renal failure are responsible.

DIARRHOEA

This is inevitable during the first few weeks but can be adequately controlled by restriction of oral fluid intake to 1,500 ml daily and by medication with Lomotil, codeine phosphate or calcium carbonate. Thirst can be troublesome, as drinking large quantities of fluids has a strong purging effect. It can often be quenched by sucking ice. Avoidance of fatty and bulky foods is also helpful.

By 6 months, stool frequency is usually diminished to an average of 2–3 times daily but, from time to time, dietary indiscretion, enteric infection or inappropriate antibiotic therapy may evoke relapse. This is often associated with anal soreness, fissure or haemorrhoids, which can be quite troublesome. Cholecyst-jejuno-ileal bypass appears to be beneficial in reducing the frequency of diarrhoea by allowing absorption of bile salts in the excluded ileum (Hallberg and Homgren, 1978).

FLUID AND ELECTROLYTE DISTURBANCES

Due to excessive diarrhoea and vomiting, electrolyte disturbances may occur during the first few weeks or months. These are easily rectified by oral supplements or, if severe, intravenous repletion of potassium, calcium and magnesium. Not infrequently, late electrolyte disturbances can be found on routine biochemical follow up. Low whole body potassium is common. A low serum magnesium, though often only mildly abnormal, was seen in 41·7% of patients at five years (Baddeley, 1979a) and metabolic bone disease has been reported by Compston *et al.* (1978) in ten out of 21 patients who underwent ileo-jejunal bypass (retaining 10 cm of jejunum and 25 cm of ileum in use). Low serum zinc and copper values occasionally occur. Hyperchloraemic acidosis is an infrequent but alarming complication. Patients manifest giddiness, ataxia, headache, amnesia, muscle weakness, confusion and variable coma (DeWind and Payne, 1976). Intravenous bicarbonate infusions are effective but, as the abnormality is liable to recur, it is usually necessary to operate and to restore the integrity of the small intestine.

MALNUTRITION

Protein malnutrition has been demonstrated in 25 per cent of post-bypass patients (Shizgal *et al.*, 1979). Hypoalbuminaemia was seen in about 10% of patients (Baddeley, 1979b) being at its most frequent during the first year. This well-recognised hazard is largely due to malabsorption of essential and non-essential amino acids and has been likened to kwashiorkor (White *et al.*, 1974). After 12 to 18 months, dilatation and elongation of the jejuno-ileum in continuity occurs and, as a result of the associated improvement in absorption, weight reduction diminishes and ceases. When this adaptation does not occur, hypoproteinaemia and electrolyte deficiencies may be serious and necessitate restoration of small bowel continuity.

Other deficiencies include impaired absorption of vitamin A, B_{12} and E. Low folate values may also occur, possibly due to bacterial colonisation of the small bowel.

FATTY LIVER

Fatty infiltration of the liver is present in about 88% of massively obese persons. Following jejuno-ileal bypass, 55% of them show further fatty change, but this is usually asymptomatic. One or more serum biochemical liver function tests may become abnormal but these changes improve after weight reduction has ceased. It is probable that the increased fatty infiltration after the operation is due to protein-calorie malnutrition affecting particularly the essential lipotropic amino acids. Hence the importance of a high-protein, low-carbohydrate, low-fat diet initiated from the outset and continued for 2 years at least.

A few patients develop evidence of hepatic insufficiency which may deteriorate, with overt liver failure and death. This hazard may be due to the effects of absorbed enteric hepatotoxins, evoked by bacterial colonisation of the included and excluded small bowel, upon a liver already affected by fatty infiltration. Absorption of lithocholic acid formed in the colon by bacterial deconjugation of chenodeoxycholic acid has also been incriminated (Sherr *et al.*, 1974).

Treatment consists of intravenous amino acid infusions (Heimburger *et al.*, 1975) and an antibiotic effective against anaerobic and aerobic organisms (Baddeley, 1979b; Powell-Jackson *et al.*, 1979). If the patient relapses after an initial response, further such treatment, followed by restoration of small bowel continuity, may be required.

CIRRHOSIS

There have been several reports of micronodular cirrhosis developing one to six years after jejuno-ileal bypass (Kern *et al.*, 1973; Mangla *et al.*, 1974; Marubbio *et al.*, 1976). The incidence was highest (8·6%) in the author's series in which liver biopsy was performed annually so that early asymptomatic cirrhosis was detected (Baddeley, 1979b). Only two patients could be labelled as alcoholic, although histological examination often showed features of this type of liver disease (Brown *et al.*, 1975). Restoration of small bowel continuity was carried out in eight of the 15 patients because of deterioration; three died post-operatively in liver failure. The remainder have been maintained on a high-protein, no-alcohol dietary regimen and routine biopsies have revealed either no deterioration or, in two patients, disappearance of the cirrhosis. Restoration of normal liver histology after discontinuance of the by-pass was reported by Soyer *et al.* (1976).

URINARY CALCULI

Oxalate in the bowel is normally bound with calcium and excreted in the faeces but, in the presence of steatorrhoea, calcium binds with fatty acids and the free oxalate is absorbed. As a result, hyperoxaluria occurs and may result in calculus formation. The incidence varies from 5 to 30% in various series. Renal failure due to oxalosis has been reported in seven patients. The problem can be minimised by prescribing, from the outset, a low-oxalate, low-fat diet and by administration of calcium or antacids such as aluminium hydroxide.

GALL-STONES

There is thought to be an increased incidence of biliary calculi, especially during the first six months after jejuno-ileal bypass. There is no decisive evidence that biliary calculi are more common thereafter; obese patients are in any case more prone to gall-stones than the non-obese.

POLYARTHALGIA

This condition, which presents as migratory rheumatoid-like joint pain but with negative serology, is similar to that found in inflammatory bowel disease. It occurs in up to 16% of patients. The rapid response to Cotrimoxazole, Metronidazole or Tetracycline in two to three days suggests an infective cause, and this has been confirmed by Wands *et al.* (1976). However, antibiotic therapy is only necessary in the more severe cases, the majority simply requiring short-term analgesics.

OTHER SYMPTOMS OF BACTERIAL OVERGROWTH

Abdominal bloating or pseudo-obstruction of the colon is common after the first post-operative year. It often varies with dietary intake and perceptive patients learn how to avoid it. It can sometimes be troublesome. If so, the antibiotics already mentioned are likely to be effective but there is always the risk of loss of sensitivity in the long term.

Bypass enteropathy is mainly seen in patients who have undergone end-to-end jejuno-ileal bypass with implantation of the excluded ileum into the sigmoid colon. Colonisation of the excluded ileum results in pyrexia, abdominal pain and pneumatosis cystoides intestinalis (Passaro *et al.*, 1976). The problem can be avoided by implantation of the ileum into the transverse colon or, preferably, by using the original end-to-side jejuno-ileostomy technique.

INDICATIONS FOR RESTORATION OF
SMALL BOWEL CONTINUITY

As mentioned, hazardous liver complications and malnutrition constitute the main indications for abandoning the bypass. Other indications are excessive diarrhoea, polyarthralgia, distressing abdominal distension, renal damage, tuberculosis, and inability to cope with the problems of the bypass. 10–15% of patients develop one or more side-effects and fail to sustain satisfactory response to treatment.

The restoration of intestinal continuity is followed by the rapid disappearance of symptoms but, unfortunately, the sense of well-being is usually accompanied by a gain of weight, despite appropriate dietary advice. Simultaneous gastric plication or bypass will prevent this and this is usually offered to those judged fit enough to tolerate the double procedure.

Gastric bypass, gastric partitioning and gastric plication

These procedures are designed to reduce gastric capacity and induce early satiety, thereby compelling the patient to take a low-calorie, weight-reducing diet. They have the attraction of not interfering with nutrient absorption in the small intestine, thus avoiding the potential metabolic hazards of jejuno-ileal bypass. They are, however, technically more difficult than this operation and consequently have been less popular until recent years.

Gastric bypass was pioneered by Mason and colleagues in Iowa, U.S.A. Starting in 1966, they evolved a technique in which the stomach was transected just below the cardia, the proximal part being drained by gastro-jejunostomy and the distal part being retained defunctioned to permit restoration of gastric continuity if the need arose (Mason and Ito, 1969). Initially, satisfactory weight reduction was not achieved, vomiting and dumping were common, and the operative mortality was as high as 3%. They then tried partial transection of the stomach at the same level, with the proximal part draining into the distal part through a narrow channel. This gastroplasty technique was a failure and was abandoned. Reverting to gastric bypass, effective weight reduction was achieved subsequently by limiting the capacity of the proximal compartment to less than 100 ml and the size of the gastro-jejunostomy to 1·2 cm (Mason *et al.*, 1975).

Subsequent modifications have included gastric bypass with Roux-en-Y gastro-jejunostomy (Griffen *et al.*, 1977), gastric partitioning and gastro-jejunostomy (Alden, 1977) and gastric plication (Pace *et al.*, 1978). In the latter two techniques, the stomach is partitioned using a stainless steel stapling instrument. In the plication method the stoma between the proximal and distal parts is achieved by prior removal of three staples to leave a small channel.

Beneficial effects

Weight reduction, comparable to that of jejuno-ileal bypass, was obtained by Griffen *et al.* (1977), Hemreck *et al.* (1976) and Alden (1977), the first being a randomised study. It remains to be seen whether this satisfactory weight reduction is sustained in the long term as it may be possible for the determined patient to 'out-eat' the gastric reduction by taking frequent high-calorie meals. There is also concern that disruption of the gastric staple line may occur after plication, thus allowing overeating and weight regain.

The same benefits of weight reduction as are seen after jejuno-ileal bypass are to be expected, such as psycho-social rehabilitation, improved glucose tolerance and reduction of fasting lipids, as well as improved respiratory function and reduction of hypertension.

Mortality and morbidity

The operative mortality has now fallen to about 1%; in Alden's series, which has now reached more than 300 cases, it is nil. As in all obese patients, there is a risk of death due to respiratory problems, pulmonary embolism and myocardial infarction. The main cause of death after gastric bypass has been peritonitis due to suture line leakage but this is less likely to occur with gastric plication, in which the stomach is not opened. In 1979, Mason *et al.* reported perforation of the proximal or distal parts of the stomach in 4·7% of 863 gastric bypass operations. It was equally common in both parts of the stomach and at the anastomosis. It also affected gastroplasty patients and occurred during the first 10 post-operative days. This complication has been seen mainly since proximal capacity has been reduced below 100 ml and stoma size to 1·2 cm. It is thought to be due to obstruction of the stoma or the afferent loop by the nasogastric tube or by technical error at operation. Early recognition of the problem has dramatically reduced its mortality.

Morbidity in the early weeks is more common than after jejuno-ileal bypass, due to vomiting caused by over-eating, bile reflux or stenosis of the stoma. Stomal ulceration has occurred in 1—6% of series so far reported. Dumping was recorded as a frequent problem in earlier reports at a time when the gastro-jejunostomy stoma was made too large. On the other hand, it is very gratifying to find that the main metabolic and enteric complications associated with jejuno-ileal bypass do not occur. The hazard to the liver is much reduced; decrease in fatty infiltration occurs from the onset and liver function tests remain normal. Indeed there appear to be very few late complications of gastric surgery for obesity.

Conclusions

Good sustained weight loss can be obtained by jejuno-ileal bypass at the expense of potential metabolic and infective side effects. Gastric reduction procedures also evoke good weight reduction and have fewer complications, although some patients may be unable to cope with the frustration of their former gluttonous eating habits and thus may not be suitable for this type of procedure. Otherwise, if the weight reduction achieved in the short term is sustained, it seems that gastric reduction surgery will largely replace jejuno-ileal bypass.

References

Alden J.F. (1977) *Arch. Surg.* **112**, 799.

Baddeley R.M. (1979a). In *The Treatment of Obesity*, ed. Munro J.F. M.T.P. Press, Lancaster, p. 165.

Baddeley R.M. (1979b) *Brit. J. Surg,* **66**, 525.

Bray G.A. (1978) *Int. J. Obesity,* **2**, 270.

Bray G.A., Greenway S.L., Barry R.E., Benfield J.R., Fizer R.L., Dahns W.T., Atkinson R.L. and Schwartz A.A. (1977) *Int. J. Obesity,* **1**, 331.

Brown R.G., O'Leary J.P. and Woodward E.R. (1974) *Amer. J. Surg.* **127**, 53.

Compston J., Horton L.W.L., Laker M.F. *et al.* (1978) *Lancet,* **ii**, 1.

DeWind L.T. and Payne J.H. (1976) *J. Amer. med. Ass.* **236**, 2298.

Fielding J.W.L. and Baddeley R.M. (1978) *Brit. J. Surg.* **65**, 30.

Griffen W.O., Young V.L. and Stevenson C.C. (1977) *Ann. Surg.* **186**, 500.

Hallburg D. and Holmgren U. (1978) *Acta chir. scand.* Suppl. **482**, 31.

Heimburger S.L., Steiger E., Gerfo P.L. *et al.* (1975) *Amer. J. Surg.* **129**, 229.

Hermreck A.S., Jewell W.R. and Hardin C.R. (1976) *Surg. Gynec. Obstet.* **80**, 498.

Kern W.H., Heger A.H., Payne J.H., DeWind L.T. (1973) *Arch. Path.* **96**, 342.

Mangla J.C., Hoy W., Kim Y. and Chopek M. (1974) *Gastroenterology,* **19**, 759.

Marubbio A.T., Buchwald H., Schwartz M.Z. and Varco R.L. (1976) *Amer. J. clin. Path.* **66**, 684.

Mason E.E. and Ito G. (1969) *Ann. Surg.* **170**, 329.

Mason E.E., Printen K.J., Hartford C.E. and Boyd W.C. (1975) *Ann. Surg.* **182**, 405.

Mason E.E., Printen K.J., Barron P., Lewis J.W., Kealey G.P. and Blommers T.J. (1979) *Ann. Surg.* **190**, 158.

Pace W.G., Martin E.W., Tetirick T. *et al.* (1978) *Ann. Surg.* **190**, 392.

Passaro E., Drenick E. and Wilson S.E. (1976) *Amer. J. Surg.* **131**, 169.

Payne J.H. and DeWind L.T. (1969) *Amer. J. Surg.* **118**, 141.

Powell-Jackson P.R., Maudgal D.P., Sharp D. *et al.* (1979) *Brit. J. Surg.* **66**, 772.

Scopinaro N., Gianetta E., Civalleri D. *et al.* (1979) *Brit. J. Surg.* **66**, 613.

Scott H.W., Sandstead H.H., Brill A.B. *et al.* (1971) *Ann. Surg.* **174**, 560.

Scott H.W., Dean R.H., Shull H.J. *et al.* (1977) *Surg. Gynec. Obstet.* **145**, 661.

Sherr H.P., Nair P.P., White J.J. *et al.* (1974) *Amer. J. clin. Nutr.* **27**, 1369.

Shizgal H.M., Forse R.A., Spanier A.H. and McClean L.D. (1979) *Surgery,* **86**, 60.

Soyer M.T., Ceballos R. and Aldrete J.S. (1976) *Surgery,* **79**, 601.

Wands J.R., Lamont J.T., Mann E. and Isselbacher K.H. (1976) *N. Engl. J. Med.* **294**, 121.

White J.J., Moxley R.T., Pozefsky T. and Lockwood D.H. (1974) *Surgery,* **75**, 829.

Chapter 25

Partial ileal bypass for hyperlipidaemia

J. I. MANN AND EMANOEL C. G. LEE

Familial hypercholesterolaemia (F.H.) is associated with a poor prognosis. Sixty per cent of male heterozygotes have had a myocardial infarction by the age of 50 years and 50% are dead by the age of 60. Monozygotes have usually died before they are 30. Because partial ileal bypass is known to lower the level of blood cholesterol, this operation has been recommended for patients who do not respond to diet or lipid-lowering drugs. However, as yet there is no conclusive evidence that lowering the blood cholesterol improves the prognosis.

Rationale of the operation

The two-fold rationale of the operation is reduction in the absorption of cholesterol by the small intestine and prevention of the re-absorption of bile acids which normally occurs in the terminal ileum. Their entero-hepatic recirculation is thereby interrupted and the catabolism of cholesterol to bile acids within the liver increased by removal of the negative feed back. Though these effects are accompanied by an increase in hepatic cholesterol synthesis, the net result is usually a sustained fall in the plasma cholesterol concentration (Boyd and Percy-Robb, 1971).

Surgical technique

Early animal studies by Buchwald and Varco (1964) and by Scott and his colleagues (1966) led to the introduction of an ileal bypass operation for hyperlipidaemia. Figure 25.1 illustrates the operation. After examination of the peritoneal cavity to exclude pathology, a careful

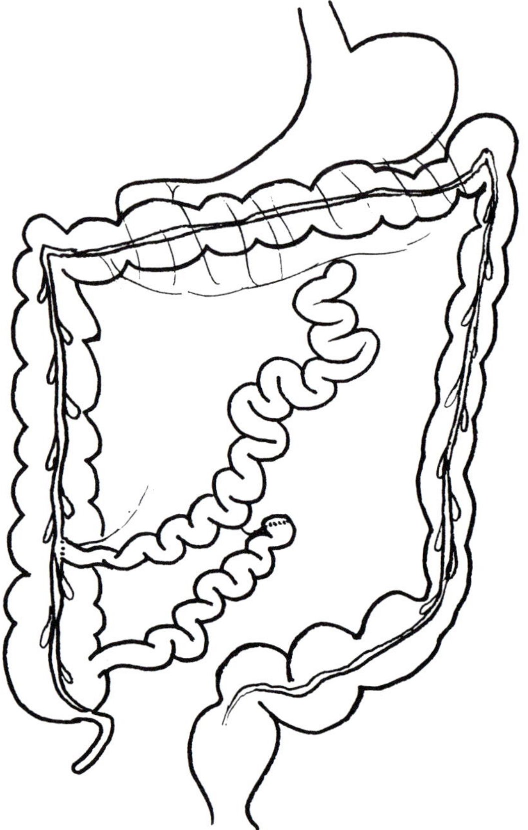

Fig. 25.1. *Partial ileal bypass.*

measurement of the small bowel is carried out from the duodeno-
jejunal flexure to the ileo-caecal valve. This is best performed by
matching a length of tape to the antimesenteric border of the intestine.
By measuring the length of the tape with a sterile metal ruler, it is
possible to obtain an accurate measurement of the length of the bowel.
The gut is then divided at the junction of middle and distal thirds. In
practice the lower ileum usually measures about 200 cms. The
proximal cut end is then anastomosed end-to-side to the caecum above
the ileo-caecal valve. The proximal end of the distal ileum is closed and
fixed to the caecum or mesentery to prevent intussusception of the
defunctioned segment.

The experience of Buchwald

The operation has been extensively employed by Buchwald and his colleagues in Minnesota. Their major review in 1974 describes 101 consecutive cases followed for at least 6 years, although about twice this number have now had the operation (Buchwald *et al.*, 1974). Impressive and sustained falls in cholesterol levels have been observed in the majority of patients, 80% having reductions in excess of 25%. The series included patients with various types of primary endogenous hyperlipidaemia (types IIa, IIb, III, and IV), and most of them also showed a fall in triglyceride levels. Patients with type IIa, however, showed an increase in triglyceride levels. Three patients with homozygous type II (familial hypercholesterolaemia) also showed substantial cholesterol reduction. Xanthomas tended to regress.

The operation appears to be safe: three cases of small-bowel obstruction have occurred, but there have been no deaths attributable to the surgical procedure. No appreciable changes have occurred in electrolytes, liver function tests or body weight. B_{12} absorption has of course been greatly reduced, but after 12 months there appears to be recovery. (Replacement therapy has invariably been given.) Alteration in bowel habit has not proved to be a problem. Most patients report that they have soft loose stools more frequently than pre-operatively, but only 20% report more than 5 stools per day. A qualitative increase in faecal fat occurs, but the only measurable consequence of this has been an occasional reduction in serum carotene. Only one patient in the series developed gallstones but it should be pointed out that 17 had had a cholecystectomy either before or during the bypass.

There is no conclusive clinical evidence that the operation is beneficial. The fact that the patients who preoperatively were free from angina remained so for at least 6 years after the operation and 70% of those with angina showed at least some improvement means little in the absence of control information. Some 30 patients had arteriography before and after surgery. Fewer than one-third showed signs of deterioration and in about 20% there was some suggestion of improvement. Although this observation is also uncontrolled, a number of published series of sequential coronary angiograms have suggested a higher rate of progression in patients not on aggressive lipid-lowering therapy. However, perhaps the most encouraging finding is that approximately three-quarters of the patients with pre-existing coronary artery disease were alive five years after the operation. The principal disadvantage of this series is the fact that the patients were suffering from a wide range of lipid disturbances, some with a prognosis not as gloomy as that of F.H. and some (for example those with a diagnosis of type III) who might have been expected almost without exception to respond to diet or simple hypolipidaemic drug therapy. Nevertheless, other large series of patients of comparable age with previous myocardial infarction suggest that, regardless of lipid disturbance, only around half are alive five years later.

Impressive controlled studies have been carried out in rhesus monkeys showing that partial ileal bypass is able to protect against the atherogenic effect of a very high cholesterol diet and also that the aortic atheroma induced by such a diet is reversed by the operation (Scott, 1978).

Experience in Oxford and elsewhere

No other large series of cases have been published. In Oxford and elsewhere small numbers of patients have had the operation (Helsingen and Rootwelt, 1969; Swan and McGowan, 1968; Sodal *et al.*, 1970). It has been our practice to consider for this operation only patients with severe heterozygous type II hyperlipoproteinaemia who are refractory to drugs or unable to tolerate them. In our experience this represents approximately 8% of the patients with familial type II hyperlipoproteinaemia referred to our Clinic. The operations have been carried out without complications and we too have observed regression of xanthomas and apparent clinical improvement. A major problem arises if coronary angiography is routinely carried out pre-operatively since a substantial proportion of such patients are likely to have major occlusions which are considered to warrant coronary artery surgery. In such cases we have recommended that this be carried out first, and the partial ileal bypass six to twelve months later.

In order to evaluate this procedure, we hope to embark on a randomized clinical trial in which patients who fail to respond to usual lipid-lowering therapy are randomized either to a group who will be advised to have surgery or to another group who will be advised to continue on medical treatment. In view of the usual outcome of the disease it is likely that definitive data will emerge from the study of a relatively small number of patients.

Portacaval shunt and hyperlipidaemia

This operation, which was pioneered by Starzl in Denver, Colorado (Starzl *et al.*, 1978), has been recommended to patients with homozygous type II hyperlipoproteinaemia and more than 30 operations are known to have been carried out. The procedure certainly produces reduction of cholesterol and fairly rapid regression of xanthomas. There is also evidence of reversal of aortic stenosis associated with the condition. Experiments in dogs have suggested that decreased hepatic cholesterol synthesis occurs when the liver is deprived of insulin. No cases of hepatic encephalopathy or deranged liver function tests have been reported but in one patient who died there was evidence of shrinkage of hepatocyte size, depletion of rough endoplasmic reticulum and the accumulation of intracytoplasmic lipid deposits in comparison with a pre-operative biopsy specimen. It is at present generally agreed that this procedure should be reserved for the rare homozygous form of type IIa hyperlipoproteinaemia.

References

Boyd S.G. and Percy-Robb I.W. (1971) *Am. J. Med.* **51**, 580.
Buchwald H., Moore R.B. and Varco R.L. (1974) *Circulation,* **49**, suppl. 1.
Buchwald H. and Varco R.L. (1964) *Surg. Forum,* **15**, 289.
Helsingen N. and Rootwelt K. (1969) *Nordisk Medicin,* **82**, 1409.
Scott H.W. (1978) *Arch. Surg.* **113**, 62.
Scott H.W., Stephenson S.E. and Younger R.K. (1966) *Ann. Surg.* **163**, 795.
Sodal G., Gjertsen, K.T. and Schrumpf A. (1970) *Acta chir. scand.* **136**, 671.
Starzl T.E., Putnam C.W., Koep L.J. (1978) *Arch. Surg.* **113**, 71.
Swan D.M. and McGowan J.M. (1968) *Amer. J. Surg.* **116**, 22.

Index